Health Care in a Changing Setting:
the UK experience

*The Ciba Foundation for the promotion of international cooperation in
medical and chemical research is a scientific and educational charity established by
CIBA Limited – now CIBA-GEIGY Limited – of Basle. The Foundation operates independently
in London under English trust law.*

*Ciba Foundation Symposia are published in collaboration with
Elsevier Scientific Publishing Company, Excerpta Medica, North-Holland Publishing Company,
in Amsterdam.*

Elsevier/Excerpta Medica/North-Holland, P.O. Box 211, Amsterdam

Health Care in a Changing Setting: the UK experience

Ciba Foundation Symposium 43 (new series)

1976

Elsevier · Excerpta Medica · North-Holland

Amsterdam · Oxford · New York

© *Copyright 1976 Ciba Foundation*

ISBN Excerpta Medica 90 219 4048 5
ISBN American Elsevier 0-444-15209-1

Published in June 1976 by Elsevier/Excerpta Medica/North-Holland, P.O. Box 211, Amsterdam, and
American Elsevier, 52 Vanderbilt Avenue, New York, N.Y. 10017.

Suggested series entry for library catalogues: Ciba Foundation Symposia
Suggested publisher's entry for library catalogues: Elsevier/Excerpta Medica/North-Holland.

Ciba Foundation Symposium 43 (new series)

Library of Congress Cataloging in Publication Data

Symposium on UK Health Needs in a Changing Setting,
    Ciba Foundation, 1975.
    Health care in a changing setting.

    (Ciba Foundation symposium ; 43 (new ser.))
    Includes bibliographical references and index.
    1.   Medical care--Great Britain--Congresses.
2.   Great Britain--National Health Service--Con-
gresses.   I.   Title.   II.   Series: Ciba Foundation.
Symposium ; 43 (new ser.)   [DNLM: 1.   Health ser-
vices--Great Britain--Congresses.   W3 C161F v. 43
1975 / W84 FA1 S9h 1975]
RA395.G6S93 1975   362.1'0941   76-15417
ISBN 0-444-15209-1 (American Elsevier)

Printed in The Netherlands by Mouton & Co, The Hague

Contents

Participants

Symposium on *UK Health Needs in a Changing Setting*, held at the Ciba Foundation, London, 3rd and 4th December 1975

Chairman: H. BRIDGER   The Tavistock Institute of Human Relations, The Tavistock Centre, Belsize Lane, London NW3 5BA

M. L. J. ABERCROMBIE   2 Bridge Lane, Little Shelford, Cambridgeshire CB2 5HE

T. H. D. ARIE   Goodmayes Hospital, Ilford, Essex IG3 8XJ

H. BADERMAN   Department of Medicine, University College Hospital, Gower Street, London WC1E 6AU

R. BECKHARD   Sloan School of Management, 5050 Memorial Drive, Cambridge, Massachusetts 02138, USA

M. BICKERTON   The Divisional Health Office, North West District, 62–74 Victoria Street, St. Albans, Hertfordshire AL1 3SZ

J. L. T. BIRLEY   Institute of Psychiatry, De Crespigny Park, Denmark Hill, London SE5 8AF

R. F. CARTER   Operational Research Service, Department of Health and Social Security, 151 Great Titchfield Street, London W1P 8AD

E. GOLLAN   Kentish Town Health Centre, 2 Bartholomew Road, London NW5 2AJ

R. GOULSTON   Stockwell Group Practice, Buckmaster House, Stockwell Park, London SW9 0UB

K. ELLIOTT   The Ciba Foundation, 41 Portland Place, London W1N 4BN

A. GUZ   Department of Medicine, Charing Cross Hospital Medical School, Fulham Palace Road, London W6 8RF

L. HOCKEY   Nursing Research Unit, Department of Nursing Studies, University of Edinburgh, 12 Buccleuch Place, Edinburgh EH8 9JT

P. J. HUNTINGFORD   Joint Academic Unit of Obstetrics, Gynaecology and Reproductive Physiology, The London Hospital Medical College, Turner Street, London E1 2AD and The Medical College of St. Bartholomew's Hospital, London EC1A 7BE

G. JOYSON   The Royal Marsden Hospital, Fulham Road, London SW3 6JJ

J. J. KNOX   Islington Community Health Council, Liverpool Road Hospital, Liverpool Road, London N1 0QE

R. LEVITT   CHC News, King's Fund Centre, 24 Nutford Place, London W1H 6AN

C. J. LUCAS   Student Health Centre, University College London, 3 Gower Place, London WC1E 6BN

M. E. McCLYMONT   Department of Social Science, Stevenage College of Further Education, Marks Wood Way, Stevenage, Hertfordshire SG1 1LA

L. H. W. PAINE   The Bethlem Royal Hospital, Monks Orchard Road, Beckenham, Kent BR3 3BX

C. J. ROBERTS   Welsh National School of Medicine, Department of Community Medicine, Heath Park, Cardiff CF4 4XN

A. D. ROY   Department of Surgery, The Queen's University of Belfast, Institute of Clinical Science, Grosvenor Road, Belfast BT12 6BJ

E. M. RUSSELL   Department of Community Medicine, University of Aberdeen, University Medical Buildings, Fosterhill, Aberdeen AB9 2ZD

I. G. TAIT   Danes House, Lee Road, Aldeburgh, Suffolk IP15 5HG

R. D. WEIR   Department of Community Medicine, University of Aberdeen, University Medical Buildings, Fosterhill, Aberdeen AB9 2ZD

Editors: RUTH PORTER *(Organizer)* and DAVID W. FITZSIMONS

Chairman's introduction

HAROLD BRIDGER

The Tavistock Institute of Human Relations, The Tavistock Centre, London

All conferences depend to one degree or another on the relevance of the themes and on the quality of the contributions and participants. The Ciba Foundation has always taken serious note of these three parameters and assured the importance of the event itself and the scientific as well as social centrality of the published product. The conference method has been traditional but has fully allowed for freedom of thought and controversy.

We meet on a topic chosen some little time ago and there is certainly no doubt about its relevance and timeliness; we are conferring in just the turbulent, complex uncertain environment where UK health and the National Health Service are seriously threatened from within and from without. Reality demands that we take note of the conditions and critical problems which face us. We must also take note of the thought-provoking papers which have been prepared for us and which we shall want to explore with their authors. We have all too little time for doing justice to these contributors and their work. How can we best reconcile these factors and forces which are present with us today?

If we go for a low-risk event we could pretend that the programme was taking place in a strongly bounded and supported health system which we can control and coordinate internally and externally. We should also, during discussion periods, concentrate entirely on exploring the papers, their contents and implications for certain developments, current or future.

A greater risk would be taken if we were to accept the reality of the environment in which we are conducting this symposium, recognized the disruptive forces besetting this meeting and acknowledged their presence in this chamber as well as outside it. On the other hand, we must not use these forces as an excuse to take flight from the primary purpose of this symposium—which is to improve our *understanding* as a necessary precondition for moving towards a sounder appreciation of the underlying forces and concomitants affecting UK health needs. All too readily both politicians and professionals succumb to the attractions of conflict round tactical 'Hill 60s' rather than confront multiple and interdependent frames of reference which require different designs and strategies.

Only in this way can we hope to prepare the options, make the choices and take the decisions which may remedy the nightmare quality of a malfunctioning reorganized National Health Service and the unhappily locked conflictual struggle of professional and political protagonists rending our national well-being in mutually destructive ways.

In agreement with Dr Ruth Porter, who organized this symposium, and after appropriate sounding and consultation with many members of this group, we shall endeavour to fulfil both the original purpose of this symposium and face the reality of the industrial strife—strikes—occurring in the health services in the UK at present. I propose that we continue to focus our attention on the papers which, independently and in concert, may well lead us to that *understanding* which is critical for considered action rather than anxiety-driven ineffectual reactions. But, after clarification and discussions of the papers themselves, I propose that discussants feel that they have both sanction and opportunity to explore the implications deriving from any one paper—or from that paper in conjunction with others—for the present and future of the National Health Service.

In this respect some papers may bear more immediately than others on the issues, but *all* will yield essential interrelated data for our better understanding. We also need to remember that during the next two days we are a *learning institution* as much concerned with the longer term as with the present—and with prevention and not only remedial efforts.

Never was the interdependence of the organic whole of the UK health picture better demonstrated than by reading through even the brief summaries of the papers that will be presented. At the same time the higher-risk element will be evidenced in the wider terms of reference which we can give ourselves as discussants.

The difficulties of changing

M. L. J. ABERCROMBIE

Little Shelford, Cambridge (and formerly Bartlett School of Architecture, University College London)

Abstract　In general, our psychological equipment develops in such a way that we get information of predictive value through the senses; we tend to record constancies and consistencies of events and behave as though these are persistent. We are mostly unaware of the power of the stores of relevant experience (assumptions, expectations, attitudes) that condition our perceptions and therefore cannot question them, nor in many circumstances is there need to do so. In fairly constant conditions they are useful in helping us to see, quickly and effortlessly, what we expect to see. But in rapid changes this is not so; we can no longer rely on our psychological equipment and we become uncertain, confused and, in extreme cases, antagonistic, fearful and impotent. Examples of assumptions that influence medical education and medical treatment are given. Ability to respond effectively to change requires confidence to examine and restructure basic assumptions. The value of interaction in small groups in helping to achieve this is indicated.

Our difficulties in accepting change are an inevitable consequence of our outstanding success, as a species, in learning to behave effectively in a fairly constant environment. In general, our psychological equipment develops in such a way that the information we receive from the environment is of predictive value. When we look at a common apple, we know just how far to stretch out a hand to reach it, how heavy it will be, how hard to the bite, how sweet, what it will smell like and even how long it will keep fresh in the refrigerator or in the warmth of the sitting room. But we can only do this if it is a common apple, a familiar variety; we cannot be so clever and accurate about a new kind. We tend to record constancies or consistencies in the sensory input and bring this store of information to every act of perception. The eye is never innocent, like the camera which has no memory.

　We are usually unaware of these expectations or assumptions and of the part they play in enabling us to get valid information easily and swiftly, in familiar conditions, and in ensuring that we fail to do so, and suffer from observer error, in new or changed conditions. Their prevalence and power can be demonstrated visually by, for instance, the rotating trapezoidal window.[1] This is a piece of cardboard cut and painted to look like a window frame seen in perspective. It is mounted on a rotating spindle fixed to the middle of the bottom edge. What most people see when they look at the rotating trapezoid is a window swinging back and forth to right and to left, as though on a hinge at the back. When a rod is placed in the window it seems to swing independently of the frame; it moves at right angles to it, then becomes closely pressed against it, and at some point or other it gets to the other side of the frame. It seems to do this in various ways; sometimes the rod elongates and bends and twists round the frame; sometimes it breaks through the frame and, occasionally, people *hear* it break through the frame! When a little red cube is stuck on a corner of the window the cube seems to move independently of the window; it may appear to slide up and down it or leave the plane of the window and circle it like a satellite. The explanation of these errors of observation is that we attribute to the trapezoidal piece of cardboard, which is painted to look like a window, all the properties of a rectangle—most windows are rectangular. The industrialized environment is full of rectangular shapes, and from birth we are surrounded by them, but a rectangle is seldom normal to the line of vision; it is much more often at an angle, so that the image it throws on the eye is trapezoidal, having a longer side nearer to us and a shorter side further away. When we look at this thing which is *actually* a trapezoid (a comparatively rare shape) and which also throws a trapezoidal image on the retina, we assume that it is a rectangle seen in perspective, and this could be the case only if the short side always remained at the back. As the window goes round and round, the short side comes to the front, but it *seems* to remain at the back, conforming to our expectations of the way rectangles behave—that is, the window is seen to be swinging backwards and forwards and not rotating. Unconsciously, we are using our experience that both rectangles and trapezoids throw trapezoidal images on the eye; but, as rectangles are much more common than trapezoids, we assume that the trapezoidal image is thrown by a rectangle, and see it as such. The assumption is so strong that it is possible to look at the trapezoid until we are blue in the face and never see it as anything but a window swinging backwards and forwards. But we can easily understand its nature by changing our position relative to it; by standing above it, or having it tilted towards us we can see that it is in fact going round and round. The illusion depends on our fixed position; take a different standpoint and we see it as it really is. Or add some contradictory evidence: when the rod or cube is put on, we see that there is something odd about the set-up, though we tend to see the rod and cube doing funny things rather than the window. If the window is loaded with several such things which challenge our assumption, the illusion may disappear. Or if we focus attention on one spot, say one corner or the junction with the spindle, we may, as it were, ignore the whole window and avoid using our assumption as to its shape.

Our tacit assumption that significant conditions remain constant can be illustrated further by the photograph of the boiler of a battleship (Fig. 1). Here we see the cylindrical boiler with rows of convex rivets joining the plates together and large irregular concavities, dents made by shell fire. If the photograph is turned upside down, the rivets become dents and the dents blisters. This is because we are accustomed to having light coming from above and have learned to interpret a shape with a shadow at the top as concave, and one with shadow below as convex. We can discover our assumption by changing the position of the object relative to ourself.

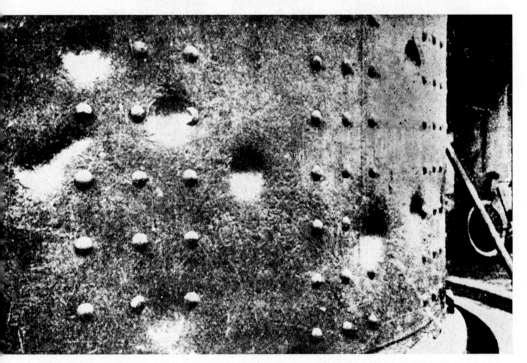

FIG. 1. Boiler of a battleship from F.H. Adler (1949) *Physiology of the Eye*, C.V. Mosby, St. Louis.

Assumptions can be revealed by comparing different people's perception of the same thing. A doctor engaged in a health education campaign to improve diet in an undeveloped region was asked by a tribesman 'But why do white men eat babies?'. White men eat many things out of tins. A tin of tomatoes may have a picture of tomatoes on the label, a tin of beef, a bull's head; there develops an assumption of consistency between the picture and the contents. But a tin with a baby's face on it does not contain a baby, only food fit for babies.

The power of the old can be seen clearly when we try to make something new. Our distant ancestors, when they first learnt to make pots of clay, put marks on them like those of basket work, or of leather thongs, according to their earlier vessels made of woven plant fibres or of animal skins. Our earliest electric car looked like a horse-drawn cab (Fig. 2). An early painting by Picasso, a supreme innovator, looked like a painting by a Pre-Raphaelite. (When he painted this picture Picasso was a devoted admirer of Burne-Jones.) (Fig. 3.)

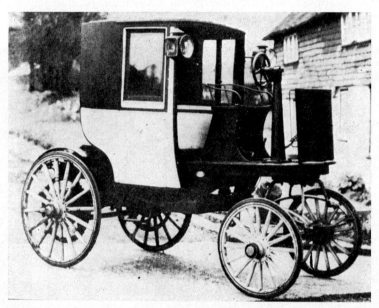

FIG. 2. Bersey Electric Cab 1897, plate 5 in P. Sumner (1969) *Motor Cars up to 1930*, Science Museum Illustrated Booklet, HMSO, London (British Crown Copyright. Science Museum, London).

Assumptions about the nature of the physical world are built up as a result of continual interaction with it. If we often fail to get valid information because things vary or change, our assumptions become modified to fit. So we gradually learn to use decimal coinage; or to behave less clumsily in the overhauled administration of the National Health Service. Adaptation to change requires *unlearning* as well as learning. There are at least two reasons why we cannot teach old dogs new tricks; because the long-term memory store is so full, there

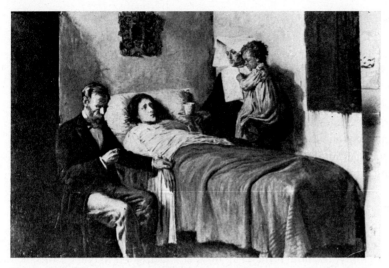

FIG. 3. *Science and Charity* (1896) by Picasso (copyright Editorial Gustavo Gili, S.A., Barcelona).

is a lot to forget and, because short-term memory weakens with age, there is less chance of new events getting into the long-term store.

But some of our assumptions, those concerned more with values and ideas than tangible physical things, are not so easily tested, corrected and refined by feedback. One of these is the commonly held idea that illness is a punishment for wrongdoing. A summary of the results of public opinion surveys on causation of cancer[2] states that 15–20% of people believed that cancer was connected with immorality. A snatch of conversation between two characters in Solzhenitsyn's *Cancer Ward*[3] illustrates how one of them ponders on the possible mechanisms of cancer control and in so doing finds a rational basis to support the belief that cancer is related to guilt, while the other, less sophisticated one who needs no such support from science, recognizes his sins and feels that they have doomed him hopelessly: ' "So I wouldn't be surprised" Kostoglotov continued, "if in a hundred years' time they discover that our organism excretes some kind of caesium salt when our conscience is clear, but not when it's burdened, and that it depends on this caesium salt whether the cells grow into a tumour or whether the tumour resolves." Yeffrem sighed hoarsely "I've mucked so many women about, left them with children hanging round their necks. They cried ... mine'll never resolve." '

It is easy to see how such beliefs prevent people from seeking medical aid, or discourage them from taking any steps to prevent cancer; to do so, with their intrapsychic set up, would be illogical.

Two basic assumptions about the role of the doctor deeply affect his educa-tion and are resistant to change because, like primitive beliefs about causation of disease, they are not easily open to test: (i) the concept that the doctor is one who *does something* to an inert patient and (ii) the idea that his education should be based on the natural sciences. I shall speak of 'the doctor', but I mean all people concerned with curing the sick.

Crudely, the doctor is seen as a person who makes a sick person well. In pre-scientific days he could do this from a distance, invoking other powers through spells, but more usually nowadays he relies on direct physical interven-tion, adding things to the body (chemicals) or subtracting bits from it (operating and, not so long ago, bleeding) or, if sufficiently open to oriental culture, sticking pins in and waggling them about. The patient is preferably inert, for an active one is not always active in the right direction; he may accept the gift of a bottle of medicine, but not swallow the correct dose at the right time; lots of bottles are left half empty, as though the drug does as much good magic on the shelf as in the body. In hospital, the extreme of regression is encouraged by taking away the patient's clothes. Listen again to Solzhenitsyn. *Cancer Ward* was staffed with most erudite, highly skilled, utterly devoted doctors. A patient arguing with one of them about his treatment says: ' "You see, you start from a completely false position. No sooner does a patient come to you than you begin to do all his thinking for him. After that, the thinking's done by your standing orders ... And once again I become a grain of sand, just like I was in the camp. Once again nothing *depends* on me." '

Related to this concept of the doctor as an all powerful external agent is his initial training in the natural, as distinct from human, sciences. Chemistry, physics and biology, but not sociology or psychology, were and commonly still are prerequisites for entry to medical training, and the study of anatomy, physiology and biochemistry commonly still precedes any contact with patients. Generally, in the premedical and preclinical years the teachers are not medically qualified or, if they are, they have opted out of medical practice. Generally, clinical education is based on the hospital, the patients seen in isolation from their natural physical and social environment. Treatment by the application of technology is emphasized, and the essentially social nature of man is tacitly ignored. For instance, the prospectus of a medical school which recently revised its curriculum was lavishly illustrated with photographs; of some 30 most were of impressive buildings and well equipped laboratories. Two photographs did include patients; in one a patient was being interviewed by a student to get material for the student's research thesis and in the other a patient was prone on a couch, all wired up to receive electroconvulsive therapy. Doctors are conditioned for work in hospitals. It is not surprising that, even in the under-

developed countries whose medical ethos is adopted from that of the industrialized West, it is difficult to get doctors to work in community medicine.

The assumption that treatment and prevention of disease must be based on
natural science has served us magnificently, facilitating the control of many
infectious and deficiency diseases. But it has not got us far enough with diseases
that are largely self-induced. It has not stopped people over-eating, or smoking,
or worrying, or driving dangerously. The doctor cannot cure such death-dealing
habits by putting things into the body or taking things out. It is the difficulties
of personal change, of learning and unlearning that have to be tackled. For
each person there is an idiosyncratic tangle of unrecognized and therefore
unquestionable assumptions at the root of his disease. Becoming well is a
change to which some are resistant.

Consider the difficulties of persuading more mothers to breast-feed their
babies. Acceptance of the medical evidence (in the sense of being able to act on
it) that breast-fed babies on the whole do better than bottle-fed babies is hindered
by an obstinate web of interrelated, mutually supporting assumptions. Some of
these can be articulated, many are below awareness: social taboos about
exposure of the body; preference for civilized over primitive, animal habits;
squeamishness about physical contact; urge to preserve the integrity of the
body; feelings about one's relationship to this one-time submissive endo-
parasite, now an aggressive demanding ectoparasite; perhaps the need to believe
that no harm could have come of it if one had been bottle-fed or had bottle-fed
another infant. No wonder the sale of baby foods goes up and up, and gives the
black man good reason to think the white man eats babies.

It is not, however, my intention to end on this note of gloom. There are
plenty of signs that medical education is moving in the right direction, towards
humanizing the curriculum and recognizing the layman as a necessary partici-
pant in treatment and prevention of sickness, his own and other people's and I
will make one further point, about the potentialities of discussion groups for
facilitating change.

When looking at the rotating trapezoid some of us probably felt slightly
uneasy, disconcerted, even physically uncomfortable, perhaps a little seasick.
More profound or significant changes from the familiar may result in confusion,
disorientation, even panic and impotence. Some experiments by Harlow[4]
are relevant to our understanding of how to cope with change.

Harlow reared baby monkeys on two sorts of substitute mothers, both models
made of wire but one was covered with terry-towelling which made it more
comfortable to cuddle than the wire one. In some experiments the young
monkeys had only a wire mother, in other only a terry-cloth mother, but the
most interesting cases were the 'dual-reared' ones, that is, they were suckled

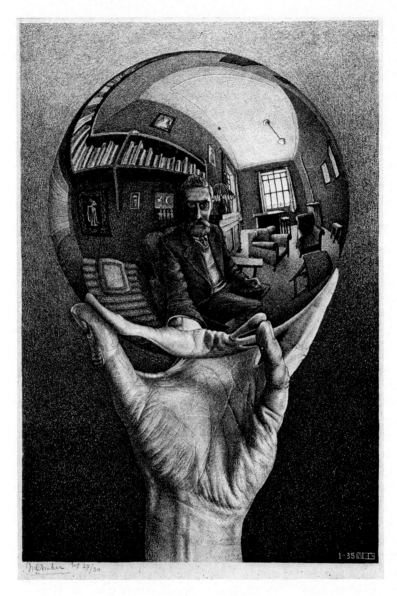

FIG. 4. *Hand with reflecting globe* by M.C. Escher (reproduced by permission of the Escher Foundation—Haags Gemeentemuseum—The Hague).

on a wire mother, but had a terry-cloth mother, without milk, available to cuddle. The young monkeys reacted differently according to their upbringing and the presence of the mother to frightening situations, such as being confronted with a mechanically moving toy animal or being put in a strange room. Monkeys brought up with a wire mother only, whether she was present or not, appeared to be too terrified by the new experience to take any interest in it, and huddled away in a corner refusing to look. Dual-reared monkeys behaved similarly unless the terry-cloth mother was present; then they would rush to her and, seeming to take comfort and security from contact with her, would turn and look back at the terrifying thing, or be able to explore the strange room. They would cuddle up to her, and make sudden expeditions from this home base to investigate, one after the other, the objects in the room, as a toddler might venture from its mother at a party, returning at intervals for reassurance. A feeling of security was necessary if the monkey was to learn about the strange things. In infancy and childhood, it is the presence of adults that helps us, and, as adults, we commonly look to surrogate parental figures, a doctor perhaps, powerful and caring. But we can learn to get security from peers, in small face-to-face groups, learning to become powerful and caring ourselves. When we have confidence in each other, we can begin to recognize our own assumptions by comparison and contrast with those of others and begin to evaluate their usefulness. We each live in a private world and look out from our egocentric position, as Escher illustrates in his *Hand with reflecting globe* (Fig. 4). Looking into a spherical mirror, we can see what is at the back of our head but, however much we move around with the globe, exploring new parts, we are always at the centre of the picture. Heath's cartoon (Fig. 5) amuses because it puts us in our place in a mouse's world. In another of Escher's pictures, *Three spheres II* (Fig. 6), we have an analogue of the group situation. Escher draws himself looking out from the centre of his globe, but reflections of other spheres alongside his own are pictured in his world. We can learn how others see their world and recognize our own basic assumptions just because they differ from others', and learn to adapt them if necessary. So groups help us to change by giving us security to perceive differences.

Discussion

Levitt: The analogy between physical change, illustrated by the rotating trapezoid, and social change is certainly tempting, but I must question your phrase 'observer error' which implies that we ought to perceive ambiguous objects 'correctly'. 'Visual illusion' is the term by which I was taught about the

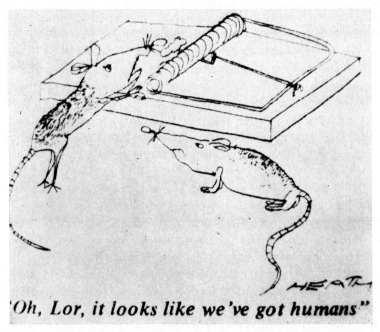

FIG. 5. Egocentric mice by Heath (1974) (reproduced by permission of *Private Eye*).

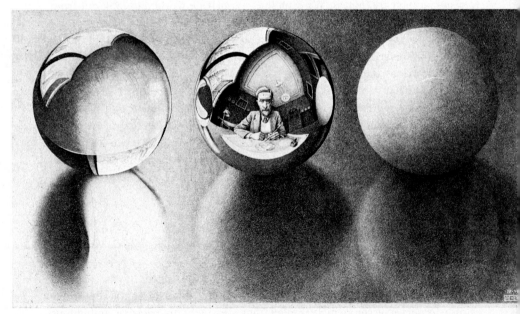

FIG. 6. *Three spheres II* by M.C. Escher (reproduced by permission of the Escher Foundation—Haags Gemeentemuseum—The Hague).

perception of ambiguous objects and it implies that either we are not provided with enough information to understand what we see or we have enough information but have not been taught how to use it. If we had studied the length of the sides of the rectangle, we would have discovered that it was a trapezoid, but you painted it like a window and so we were fooled. By calling it observer error, are you attributing conscious motivation to behaviour that is probably unconscious and involuntary?

Abercrombie: I try to avoid the term visual illusion because most things that are presented as such have no meaning for learning. I initially used this material to try to teach medical students how to see things and how to draw reasonable conclusions from what they saw. I became increasingly aware that observer error is not deliberate, in the way you imply, but an inevitable consequence of the use of experience, the use of basic assumptions, and that observer error in medicine is no different from observer error and observer skill in everyday life. One cannot teach people about it as one can about X-rays or whatever; it has to be understood within, as something that everybody has.

Roy: You have brought to our attention what we sense about our egocentricity but often tend to suppress. Can egocentricity be controlled and perhaps used to advantage?

Abercrombie: In talking about day-to-day problems in group discussions one can begin to untangle one's own basic assumptions; other people in a group see the same thing differently. Knowing that they see it through their basic assumptions, one can appreciate that one has a different set of basic assumptions. In a group, one can then compare and contrast these assumptions. I know of no other way. It is what happens during life, but more slowly and perhaps erratically. The group discussion that our chairman will probably foster will be one that offers security—the round group in which we are sitting is a secure 'nest'—and that makes one less frightened of considering alternatives.

Damage is done when the egocentricity of one person is imposed upon another; as when, for instance, a bureaucrat takes a decision in ignorance of the implications for the person affected by that decision. He is in a position of being able to abstract himself and plan, without personal experience and immediate feedback.

Joyson: Usually, subliminal techniques are used for bad purposes, but they could be channelled for good. Have you ever experienced them?

Abercrombie: No. I realize that we are influenced by things that we are not aware of. The use of subliminal perception to manipulate others at a below-awareness level seems to me wrong, however effective it may be.

Goulston: You seem to assume that the members of a group are anxious to enlarge and develop their ideas. Maybe one is comfortable with one's ideas and is terrified of change. Problems could arise if some members of a group wanted change while others were frightened of it. Is not self-awareness of the individual a basic aim that we ought to consider?

Abercrombie: The way one recruits people to a group depends on the level at which one intends to work. Some people shrink away if invited to come to a group and become self-aware, but they may come if asked to discuss current professional difficulties.

During the last three years I have been working on a project supported by the University Grants Committee to improve small group teaching in universities. Many teachers do not like the idea but some (though few) are enthusiastic. There is a general feeling that one ought to teach in small groups, but many people feel that they don't need to learn how to do so. One can only let them get on with it and help those who really want help.

Tait: You said that change is uncomfortable but could be less threatening if we felt happy and safe in a group. Although a group has to be secure to be able to change, doesn't it have to be slightly uncomfortable as well? Skill is needed in matching the discomfort to the support. When we consider changing our professional attitudes and roles in the health service we have to balance these two aspects carefully. Perhaps our recent troubles stem from the fact that we have been subjected to too much change and too little support.

Beckhard: Dr Abercrombie, if it is difficult for a child to empathize, it is difficult for an adult, too. I assume that you were implying that it is possible to increase one's functional skill through group discussion.

One problem in education is the assumption that we concentrate on training doctors and other health workers in the scientific method. Does a doctor begin to become aware of himself as a healer during his medical education rather than when he is in practice? In the USA, we are deeply concerned about whether we ought to reconstruct the clinical curriculum by adding pieces of the social curriculum to it.

Abercrombie: Many people who want to train as doctors want to treat the sick. (Some want to do research and science apart from clinical work, but these people are not part of the problem.) The doctor needs not only to empathize with the patient but also to act effectively with regard to the problem. I believe that we are all terribly handicapped—we use only a small part of our equipment. The brain is the best general computer and the cheapest, being assembled by unskilled labour. But we operate it with unskilled labour, partly because each of us is unaware of much that is inside his or her own head. What is needed is an extension of self-control, self-exploitation, self-understanding, the weaning away from inhibiting influences, and that I believe one can learn in groups. This is in addition to the better understanding of the patient that one may get from introduction of parts of the social curriculum, as you suggest. These two aspects should be closely linked in the educational process. In practice, one understands oneself better, as well as the patient, by reflection and resonance with him, just as with one's peers in the group.

Guz: I am not sure that the motivation of most students who go into medicine is to treat the sick. Although it is difficult to find the truth, informal questioning reveals motives that are horrifying (except to those who call themselves realistic): for instance, the demand for a secure living in an age in which everything is crashing. The feeling that the healer of the sick will never crash may not be true, but this is a strong motive. Another strong motive is intellectual curiosity. Nowadays, the students are often *la crème de la crème* academically (in terms of A levels, whatever they might mean). There is a certain embarrassment about talking about wanting to treat the sick. I am not condemning this, but non-medical people ought to be aware that just treating the sick is not the dominant motivation at the moment (even though it may have been in William Harvey's time). I wish it were a stronger motivation.

Bridger: The mention of curiosity rather than any other motivation gives hope that we might be more interested in prevention rather than in cure only.

Birley: Some doctors who are keen to treat the sick scare the pants off me. One can see terrible damage, certainly in psychiatry, following enthusiasm for treating the sick. This raises the questions of what we want and what we need, and what patients want and need. People should be taught when to stop treating the sick. Doctors are inclined to invent diseases which they can treat. I wonder whether Dr Abercrombie has invented the new disease of not being able to use three quarters of one's brain!

Tait: We must differentiate between treating the disease and caring for the sick. I am concerned that we now have a profession that tends to undervalue the latter role in medical education. The management of chronic and degenerative disease is the major task of doctors today. We must prepare our students for this kind of medical work.

Guz: It may sound crazy to modern medical people but there is an enormous difference between caring and treating. I agree with Dr Birley. There are classic examples in medicine where some of us continue to do what we believe is right without the slightest proof that it is the right thing to do: we stop 'clotting' with anticoagulants in myocardial infarction and yet we have no idea whether this is beneficial. Do we create some disasters in this way? Such examples multiplied many times, particularly in relation to the doctor's prescription pad, are responsible for a vast amount of iatrogenic disease. The motivating factor for prescribing drugs is not just to 'get rid of' the patient, but the desire to treat. The doctor who is told that such and such a treatment is good may not have the time to check the literature because of the pressure of work; he may not even be trained to examine the question properly. Before we reject science or push it aside, we must remember that beside the traditional laboratory aspects of medicine we must examine the validity of what we are doing with the most rigorous scientific methods. This is where we run into ethical problems; our colleagues may accuse us of being ethically wrong if we do not use a certain treatment, and they may call us 'immoral' if we claim that we know of no evidence for its efficacy. This is common nowadays. Without the rigorous discipline of science we are lost.

Abercrombie: Perhaps I oversimplified. I was trying to contrast, for example, what the student has to do 10 years after his studies with what he does in the preclinical medical course. He does not want to dissect corpses day after day; that is not a task he bought, so to speak. The preclinical course is taught by people who have opted out of *human* medicine, even if they qualified in medicine. The general attitude is pro-science and anti-human; consider, for instance, the prospectus of the medical school (p. 8). Whatever the motivation in terms of security, the job ought to be something one wants to do and something that one does well. One may have started for 'disreputable' reasons (good salary, respectable position) but one must be trained to do that job well and not to do something totally different.

Guz: In medical schools, many of us, including clinically qualified pre-clinical scientists, are exceedingly worried about the role of the preclinical sciences: their importance and the fact that they are increasingly being taught by non-medical people (because of the differences in salary). Referring to the Picasso painting (Fig. 3, p. 7), you implied that science cuts one off from charity. I deny that that is necessarily so. It is far too facile to believe that science and charity do not mix. Science has been extremely successful: 30 years ago, we learnt a medicine which was a jumble of facts, supposed or true; much of this jumble has now disappeared as the discipline of science has been brought to bear. Certainly, we cannot deal with self-induced diseases, but then we are often dealing with problems which are, conventionally, outside our competence. How do we stop smoking when the government makes a lot of its money from smoking?

Roy: In medical schools and teaching hospitals, some of us are trying to explore possibilities for change and to find solutions to some of these problems. Many of our clinical colleagues, however, think it is not appropriate that they should do so. How can we engender a spirit of enquiry into the problems facing us so that we can enter into a dialogue with our colleagues instead of being faced with blank incomprehension?

Abercrombie: Changes have taken place: 10 years ago there was little talk about small groups in teaching, but now they are fashionable. Size and numbers create barriers and a feeling that we must all march the same way, if we move at all. One must try to collect a few open-minded people already interested in the problems of medical education, and just expect that interest will grow. I realize that one cannot convert a whole medical school in a few minutes, but often the conversion takes place not within the place of teaching, but elsewhere.

Hockey: We are facing similar problems in the academic preparation of nurses for their eventual contribution to health care: we tend to put new students, who presumably are motivated to care for sick people, into an academic setting where they do not even see a patient. We have partially succeeded in overcoming this paradox in Edinburgh. For example, we put students into a wheelchair for a day and let them be taken round the city by their peers. Such experience helps them to understand a little of what it feels like to be a handicapped person. Also, in their first summer before they start their courses, we send them into geriatric units to work as auxiliaries. Perhaps if medical students were to do this, they could begin to look at matters from another viewpoint.

With regard to helping group dynamics, one should introduce someone from the other side of the fence into discussion groups which tend to consist of people who think alike—a self-selected élite. Homogeneous groups such as these are likely to be more static than dynamic.

Knox: Group development work and other tools of the social and behavioural scientist are fashionable, but we should recognize that there may be situations in which, however worthy the goals and intentions, such skills can be applied to the disadvantage of the very groups and individuals they aim to help. Social and behavioural scientists today—and in particular practitioners and investigators of behaviour change—find themselves in a situation which has many parallels to that of the nuclear scientist, bacteriologist or chemist. While our intentions may be towards ameliorating the social condition, and in the short-term seem beneficial, the long-term effects may be less clearly constructive. As Kelman has pointed out,[5] knowledge is not ethically neutral and the goodness of doing good is ambiguous. Others, notably Bradford[6] and Rogers & Skinner,[7] have questioned the assumption that the principles of group leadership—variously called applied group dynamics, human relations skills, or group process sensitivity—are necessarily congenial to democratic values. The processes are designed to involve the group in decision-making and to foster self-expression on the part of the individual member. Yet possibilities for manipulation abound, and a skilful leader may not only manipulate the group so as to get the decisions he wants, but create the feeling that these decisions reflect the will of the group discovered through the workings of the democratic process. In my own experience of community participation groups in the USA,[8] this may not result from deliberate deception on the part of the leader, who often deludes himself that he had no influence over the decision of the group. Recently, social and behavioural sciences have been introduced as part of medical school curricula. For example, H. Reicken has been developing courses at the Philadelphia Medical School and Sheila Hillier now teaches social sciences at the London and St Bartholomew's Medical Schools; their experience will be valuable. We should perhaps focus more deliberately upon ways to counteract manipulative forces and on the conditions which favour a person's ability to exercise choice and maximize his individual values.

Abercrombie: The groups with which I am concerned are not those that teach one how to manage groups but rather they are groups in which one learns how to manage oneself. One has to decide for oneself how to use—for good, for bad, or not at all—whatever power this gives one to control other people. I regard some people who call themselves 'group dynamics experts' as immoral manipulators.

Beckhard: Using a group as a forum, as a mechanism for individuals to learn and understand and improve their own behaviour in groups, is a very different matter from teaching how to lead or manage groups. These activities tend to get mixed up. It is important to distinguish the purpose of a particular training group.

Lucas: We have been speaking from the point of view of the individual with his assumptions. Individuals tend to move into groups that reinforce and support their roles and beliefs. There develops a need for interchanges between groups sharing their own sets of assumptions.

Abercrombie: This underlines the whole problem of specialization; fertilization by this cross-disciplinary work is what a symposium like this should be about.

References

[1] AMES, A. (1951) Visual perception and the rotating trapezoid window. *Psychological Monographs (General and Applied) 65*, 324–356
[2] UNION INTERNATIONALE CONTRE LE CANCER (1967) *Public Education about Cancer Monograph Series*, vol. 5, Springer Verlag, Berlin
[3] SOLZHENITSYN, A. (1968) *Cancer Ward*, Bodley Head, London
[4] HARLOW, H.F. (1959) Love in infant monkeys. *Scientific American*, June, 68–74
[5] KELMAN, H.C. (1963) Manipulation of human behaviour: an ethical dilemma for the social scientist, in American Psychological Association Symposium, American Psychological Association, Philadelphia
[6] BRADFORD, L. (1963) *Presidential Address*, in American Psychological Association Symposium, American Psychological Association, Philadelphia

7 ROGERS, C.R. & SKINNER, B.F. (1956) Some issues concerning the control of human behaviour. *Science (Washington D.C.) 124*, 1057–1066

8 KNOX, J.J. (1976) New clients for the social and behavioural sciences: helping community groups, in American Public Health Association New Orleans Conference, American Public Health Association, Washington D.C.

The reorganized National Health Service: theory and reality

LESLIE H. W. PAINE

The Bethlem Royal Hospital and The Maudsley Hospital, London

Abstract The administrative structure of the National Health Service was reorganized on 1 April 1974. The previously tripartite service—hospitals, family practitioners, local authority health services, each separately administered—was replaced by a unified structure administered by comprehensive health authorities. The Regional and/or Area Health Authorities thus appointed are designed to work under the general direction of the central departments of health to provide their populations with comprehensive integrated health care. Management on a consensus basis is undertaken by interprofessional teams of senior officers—advisory to their Authorities at the upper levels of the service and directly responsible for the administration of services at the lowest (district) level. Health authorities are conterminous as far as possible with the reformed local authorities. The consumer's voice in the reorganized Service comes from new Community Health Councils—one for every Health District.

The main aims of reorganization are presumably operational integration and better planning of services, and a more flexible use of resources for better and more comprehensive care to the individual. The main problem that the new service faced was whether it could achieve these aims and provide a more efficient and effective system of health care without at the same time introducing a stultifying and expensive bureaucracy.

Even though, admittedly, the reorganized health service is still in a state of transition, on the evidence of the first 18 months of its existence the basic problem has not been overcome and an administrative bureaucracy, in the pejorative sense of the word, has been created.

In this paper, I shall put forward some brief and somewhat random thoughts to support a general contention that the reorganization of the administrative structure of the National Health Service (NHS) in Britain, which was introduced in April 1974, is a good idea not very well executed. The introduction of the new system has not, at least in England, solved one of the 64-dollar questions about health care—how to provide adequate planning and control so that we get our priorities of provision right, without at the same time introducing the sort of bureaucracy that is inimical to any good Health Service.

I use the phrase 'in England' deliberately in order to remind you that we do not have just one National Health Service in Britain but six: England, Scotland, Wales, Northern Ireland, the Isle of Man and the Channel Islands each has its own. Even within the United Kingdom (i.e. excluding the Isle of Man and the Channel Islands) the National Health Services of Scotland and Northern Ireland were set up by separate acts of Parliament; and, though the NHS Act of 1946 originally applied to both England and Wales, the Welsh Health Service is now the responsibility of the Secretary of State for Wales working through the Welsh Office. In the same way, the central government departments concerned with health in Scotland and Northern Ireland are the Scottish Home and Health Department and the Northern Irish Department of Health and Social Services, respectively.

What I should also make clear at the outset, to ensure that there is no misunderstanding, is that, although these various services are based on the same principle, they differ slightly in the way that the principle is put into practice. Northern Ireland, for example, is the only one of the four countries in which health and social services are jointly administered by the same authority; and of the four countries only England has a regional health authority tier in its administration.

It is, therefore, not the principle but the practice of the new NHS in England that I criticize. I am in no way antipathetic to the aims of the new structure, for these, as I see them, are wholly admirable. Nobody could quarrel with the idea of integrating separate health services into a comprehensive whole so as to give better care to the individual and use resources more flexibly to redress inequalities and, in particular, the imbalance that appears to have grown up between hospital and community.

This seems to me to be not only a natural and desirable trend but one that is discernible in many other countries. All that I am saying at this juncture is that, having been the first to take a step in this particular direction, we in Britain are suffering the difficulties of innovators and should be prepared to admit this fact and learn from it.

And the first thing we should learn is that administering services is not the same as providing them. What has constantly worried me about the reorganization is the impression that it gave and still gives to many people that integrated health care will naturally flow from integrated administration. Without wishing in any way to undervalue the sort of work I and those like me do, I maintain that in the restructuring of the NHS much too much faith has been pinned on administration. Too high regard has been paid to the way health care is managed and too little to the impact this can have on the clinicians (by whom I mean the nurses, social workers, physiotherapists and others as well as the doctors). These after all are the front line troops in the battle for health and the administrators come well to the rear.

In a nutshell I am suggesting that our new system has perhaps overlooked the simple fact that patients come to health services to be treated and not administered; that the NHS is basically no more than an organization designed to deliver care and treatment as swiftly as possible to sick people; that management must be the servant of the service and not its master; and that the prime function of the administrator is to enable the clinicians to achieve their full potential in caring for the sick.

I also venture to suggest that the administrative style of the new service— management on a consensus basis undertaken by interprofessional teams—is a good one. If we are to have interprofessional health care undertaken by multi- disciplinary clinical teams, then it would appear to me to be both right and natural that the management of the services and institutions which provide that care should also be undertaken on an interprofessional basis.

What seems to have gone wrong with the new system, however, is not so much the style but the form of its administration. We have introduced into a service that should be essentially personal, humane and speedy in its action a strong element of administrative remote control which is inevitably cumber- some, expensive and slow and, therefore, highly frustrating to those who are the direct providers of care.

The four-tier structure in England (Department of Health and Social Security; Regional Health Authorities; Area Health Authorities; District Management Teams) was supposedly based on a principle of maximum delega- tion downward and maximum accountability upward. In practice, as any experienced administrator might have expected, each tier now seems to be intent, in a spirit of self-fulfilment or self-justification, on controlling rather than working with the one below it—a situation that sounds the death knell of efficient administration.

Most of those who work in the new service seem to be agreed that we have at least one too many administrative tiers in England and that as a result decision taking has been slowed down rather than speeded up since April 1974.

Admittedly, the new service is still in a state of transition. Many who are concerned with its administration are, metaphorically speaking, blundering about in the dust and chaos of what has been a great change; given time, they may be able to resolve some of the current management difficulties for them- selves. Because of this and because staff morale is now at a low ebb, I suggest that, even though an administrative tier must be removed, it might be better not to do this for some time yet—not perhaps for five years. In this respect,

as in several others (including the issue of private patients), we might be wise
to await the report of the proposed Royal Commission on the health service
before taking any action.

This does not mean that we should do nothing in the interim. The way that
the four tiers interrelate should be carefully investigated with the principle of
maximum delegation firmly in mind. The districts—those places where the
service actually meets the sick—must be allowed to get on with their jobs with
the minimum possible interference. Something also should be done about the
composition of Area Health Authorities. Although I am ready to agree that I
may be guilty of generalizing for the whole country from my particular experiences of London, the small compact Area Health Authority, consisting of
people with extensive management skills (as envisaged in the theory of reorganization), has just not materialized in practice.

Those authorities of which I have any knowledge are considerably larger than
originally envisaged; increasingly made up of local councillors because of what
the Government describes as the need to 'democratize' the Service; and involved
in too little management and too much ideological political bickering. It is time
that the NHS at all levels stopped being the butt of party politics and became
instead an interparty responsibility in the interest of the nation as a whole.

We also have a long way to go yet before the other two organizations designed
to link the administrative health authorities to the public—the Joint Consultative Committees with the local authorities, and the consumer bodies, namely
the Community Health Councils—begin to work effectively. In addition it
will be some time before the family practitioner committees are really cemented
into the new structure.

Obviously, it is early to criticize any of these bodies. But they all, and especially
the Community Health Councils, have vital roles if only we and they can decide
exactly what these should be and pursue them with vigour.

A further problem which reorganization has highlighted is the difficulty of
fitting clinicians into the management teams. With a system of interprofessional
management this problem would exist whatever administrative structure was
in being, but it is nevertheless a very real one. For let us not forget that whereas
all the various paid administrators work full time, the consultant and general
practitioner members of District Management Teams do not. Very much
part-time administrators, they also face the difficulty of trying to represent
large numbers of disparate colleagues. And yet, as I have suggested, unless
they can play their full part in the increasing number of meetings and discussions that are now taking place, then the prime function of the NHS—patient
care—is liable to lose its essential place in the foreground of all our thoughts.

As an administrator, I level a further criticism at reorganization, namely the heavy emphasis it places on the need for planning without providing effective means of doing it. Service planning, rightly, is seen as a key management function in the new service, to ensure that we achieve a proper balance of priorities between varying services and between hospital and community. But it assumes—I believe wrongly—that we have the necessary data and information upon which to base wise planning decisions. And as all planning by its very nature inhibits action, there is a great deal of truth in the proposition that our new administrative structure is good in theory for planning but bad for it in practice and even worse for management.

In Sweden, a country which is said to have the most advanced and well planned welfare state with one of the best organized health services in the world (with the minimum of private practice), the principal criticism that the public makes of the health care system is that it is inhumane, bureaucratic, slow and offers no freedom of choice. Our system in the UK is open to similar criticism, primarily because we are falling into the old trap of making the best the enemy of the good—of having too much centralization, too much planning and too much standardization, to the detriment of immediate care for the sick.

Certainly, we all seem to be spending more and more time at meetings, at working parties, liaison committees and planning groups, when perhaps we should be running our services in the best interests of the patients. This does not mean that I am against the idea of the new health care planning teams; quite the opposite—I believe they will be a key way in which the new service will be made better for the patients; as long, that is, as they remain practical rather than theoretical in their thinking. If the patients in the short term are not to suffer from too great a concentration by the providers on long-term planning then the time must come when the talking has to stop and the action has to start.

In this connection, the flight of health authority members and senior administrators of all sorts away from the hospitals and into the Area and Regional Health Authorities and the District Management Teams has meant that the most expensive element of the service, the hospitals, are now managed by some of our most junior administrators.

As the proof of any pudding is in the eating, in the end the reorganized NHS must stand or fall on its ability to show that it *is* providing better patient care. Otherwise, the considerable extra expenditure that has gone into its creation and which might have been spent directly on the patient will be wasted.

How can it demonstrate in due course that it has earned its keep? I think it can only do this by tackling some of the major issues that have faced health service policy makers since 1948. These are: the continuing and inevitable shortage of money; the shortage of manpower; and the need to establish equality in the service as a whole. So far, and naturally because of the short time that it has been in operation, the reorganized service has not shown one way or the other whether it is capable of solving these problems. But is it likely to do so and, if so, how?

In the first respect and against a background of inflation and world recession, the emphasis must be on making better use of the £4000 million or so that we at present spend on the NHS. We are unlikely to get more in real terms for some time to come, unless North Sea oil is an even greater bonanza than many at present believe. This will mean that necessity will have to be the mother of invention and, here, it must remain to be seen whether the new management will be successful or not.

With regard to the second major issue (shortage of manpower), the problems seem to be as much about maldistribution as with shortage. Overall deficiencies in medical manpower are perhaps in some respects less important than the differences which exist in the distribution between specialties and geographical locations. Considerable effort will be necessary if we are to improve distribution while retaining that basis of any good health service—a sufficient and effective corps of family doctors and general practitioners.

Finally, the problem of regional differences in the quantity and quality of care available will have to be tackled, for as one informed critic has suggested 'it remains after 25 years perhaps the most major unresolved and most baffling problem of our health care system'.

Whether reorganization can do anything about these problems it is hard to say, but I believe that if given the chance the new NHS could begin to make some headway in solving them. First, however, it must take all the necessary steps to rid itself of unnecessary bureaucracy and that will involve, *inter alia*, removing one of the present four tiers; ensuring the fullest possible delegation of responsibility and authority to the health districts; reminding health authorities of their management role and encouraging Community Health Councils to be real consumer representatives; making some arrangement whereby the doctors can have time for their administrative duties; and giving health care planning teams a chance to do their job properly by seriously setting about the collection of the necessary data for genuine service planning.

Discussion

Knox: You have suggested that the overriding problem of the reorganized NHS is 'bureaucracy' which arrived as if by magic in April 1974, but surely many of the current difficulties stem from conditions which existed long before and have progressively worsened? Doctors now have to play new and, to them, both strange and not altogether acceptable roles in health service management and planning. Doctors have traditionally exercised a degree of control over their own services which is virtually unparalleled elsewhere. They have had the authority to direct and evaluate the work of others without in turn being subject to normal direction and evaluation by them. Paradoxically, this very autonomy—embodied in the principle of full clinical freedom—is sustained by the dominance of their expertise[1] in the division of labour and resource allocation—what Freidson[2] has called 'the hierarchy of institutionalised expertise'. These attitudes to professional exclusivity tend to be infectious, as Wilson[3] demonstrated 25 years ago in his study of hospital auxiliaries: 'people tend to deal with problems of domain by attempting to limit responsibility and increase efficiency through the formulation of rules and regulations and by developing an authoritative and protective discipline'. Freidson[2] and Daniels[4] have shown that health service administrators, too, adopt similar and complementary attitudes and structures to those of their medical colleagues.

Hockey: Mr Paine, I doubt whether we are lacking data and information; masses of data on almost everything are tucked away in the archives, in medical records and elsewhere, but nobody has the skill, ability, motivation or interest to use them for planning.

Paine: Professor T. E. Chester (Manchester University) is supposed to have said 'there are millions of data untouched by human brain' and he is probably right. The difficulty lies in working the data into a system that we can use. It is not easy to appraise the effectiveness of health care: I do not know what sort of information I should need to do so.

Russell: Certainly there are far too many data but they are not in a usable form. Before we can use data for planning, we must realize that we lack measures of the effectiveness of the medical care that we are dispensing. We have impressions and short-term ideas of successes of treatment but we cannot quantitatively compare, for instance, the outcome of care of the elderly with that of care of children. Also, in our present system for the collection of routine data, we cannot identify the groups of people in the community who use specific services. We can identify who goes into hospital and why but we cannot measure how much different kinds of diseases or problems draw on the different services.

Tait: I am not clear that we yet know what we ought to measure when evaluating outcome. The right outcome as doctors conceive it may differ in many instances from the desirable outcome as the patient conceives it. Might not the Community Health Council be the kind of body that could help to clarify what patients conceive as desirable outcome? We might then have some agreed criteria for its measurement.

Russell: In any discussion with other professional groups about matters relevant to health care planning teams, every group claims that it is short of manpower and needs somebody less skilled to help it. Also, every group tries to pass what they define as the more routine tasks down the line (as they define the line). Underlying this question of what is the discrete task of every profession are issues of professionalism and job demarcation. This seems to be a critical area that must be examined carefully, because many groups are beginning to talk about the same pool of less skilled manpower in the community.

Roy: Mr Paine must defend his proposition that one tier should go but only in four or five years' time. Such a delay would be the most demoralizing prospect of all.

When clinicians are called to serve on committees they confuse their roles. They are not sure whether they are representatives or delegates. Many of our problems would be solved if clinicians would agree that when they elect one of their number to serve on a committee he is a delegate and can exercise his individual judgement, being bound by decisions to which he is a party. At present, discussions are frustrated by the fact that everybody wants his particular interest to be represented; the chosen representative is then committed to the defence of narrow interests and is almost precluded from using his innate intelligence and judgement to contribute to discussions and decision. Further, if he does not represent precisely the views of the others, then often he is disowned, leading to further trouble and confusion.

Bridger: In such intergroup situations, it is as if each individual is talking through the ghost of the group behind him and is not able to give his independent viewpoint or give appropriate weight to the institution as a whole. In this way, for example, unions and management face the same problems.

Roberts: Preoccupation with day-to-day problems in management, at this stage, may divert our attention from the objectives of reorganization and hence from some of its implications. Seemingly, reorganization is seen as the structure in which health care can best be distributed to the maximum number of people within any given set of financial constraints. It rightly follows that the primary concern of the officers of reorganization (i.e. management) is the health of the whole population (of, say, an Area Health Authority or a Regional Health Authority) and not that of individual persons within the administrative unit. However, the primary concern of nearly everyone in the medical profession has traditionally been the health of the individual patient. Reorganization and coincidental economic constraints have brought this conflict of objectives into the open. Since management has little room for manoeuvre (its goals were laid down at the inception of the National Health Service but only recently have some of the implications been appreciated), the only solution seems to be by way of a compromise which will require clinicians working in the NHS to, in part, abdicate their original historical objective (i.e. a primary concern of the health of the individual patient) and adopt one which could be said to have greater contemporary relevance, i.e. one which encompasses maximum benefit for the patient with maximum savings for the State. It is important to consider carefully the implications of such a change for both the clinician and the patient. If one of us were seriously ill, by whom would he or she prefer to be treated—a doctor whose primary objective was maximum benefit for the patient or one whose objective had swung well towards the best cost/benefit ratio for the State?

Guz: This conflict has been expressed by Mr A. Spanswick of the Confederation of Health Service Employees:[5] 'savings could be made by not buying "unnecessary equipment", such as some electronic equipment and heart–lung machines. A decision may have to be made to treat large numbers of patients rather than small numbers with unusual conditions'. With the limitation of financial resources how are we going to face this problem of cost and benefit?

Bridger: Is it simply an either/or choice? Behind this confronting issue of either/or lies the conflict of policy objectives. Would it be more practical to settle the policy first? This means putting the 'fight' further back i.e. with the Department of Health, but it will be in the right place.

Guz: But it is a confronting issue for many of us as we spend more of our time dealing with acute episodes in the chronic sick, using more and more resources and ending up with old people who are lonely, deserted by their children, poor and live in unheated homes. We have achieved these miracles with a vast use of resources. It is a terrible problem that we are all increasingly being faced with.

Bridger: That is so as long as we continue to use a system of separate limited objectives and structures in the health service more related to different sections of the Department of Health and Social Security than to a more open interdependent system. This comes back to Dr Abercrombie's point that whilst a primary objective of people coming to work in the NHS is that the service should be geared to curing the sick, it is actually structured according to the way that the Department and the management consultants they used decided. The mixture of political and conflicting limited organizational principles of doubtful relevance may not fit the basic assumptions of those working in the service—or even the tasks and problems to be tackled.

Birley: A myth which we come into contact with early is that heaven is up, hell is down, and that, on the whole, the further up we go the better we do. The same can be applied to the NHS, the structure of which can be represented by a pyramid: the higher up one is the better one is—and the better off one is. Like the natives whom Dr Abercrombie mentioned (p. 5) who were convinced that white men eat babies, I want to ask why we 'go into war backwards'? If we are going to 'do battle' in the health service, why are all the arrowheads of attack pointing away from the patient, with the most expensive points at the top of the pyramid, although the 'battle' is at the bottom, the district? One problem for any health organization is the distribution of money. It is now possible, under the reorganized system, to consider how best to spend the money within the health service of a district. Hospitals are the most expensive places for providing a health service.

Bickerton: I endorse that. I am on the battlefield at district level; the nurses are irritated and frustrated because needs are identified and discussed at district level but no further action can be taken until further discussions are held at area level by yet another team of officers not directly involved. What applies to one district does not necessarily apply to another, so that not all area decisions are applicable to every district.

One benefit for nurses from the integration of the NHS is that at last the conflict of 'us' against 'them' has been removed. For the first time, we are bringing together the community and hospitals in both of which, for years, nursing has been an entirely separate service.

References

[1] ASHFORD, J.R., FERSTER, G. & MAKUC, D. (1973) An approach to resource allocation in the reorganized National Health Service, in *The Future—and Present Indicatives*, Nuffield Provincial Hospitals Trust, Oxford University Press, London

[2] FREIDSON, E. (1970) *Professional Dominance: The Social Structure of Medical Care*, Atherton Press, New York

[3] WILSON, A.T.M. (1950) Hospital nursing auxiliaries. *Human Relations 3*, 89–94

[4] DANIELS, A. (1972) *Problems of Social Change in Control of the Professions*, Scientific Analysis Corporation, USA (unpublished essay)

[5] SPANSWICK, A. (1975) *The Times*, Nov. 25, p. 1

Changing concepts in university health

C. J. LUCAS

Student Health Centre, University College London

Abstract Some of the underlying concepts and models which have influenced the provision of health care in university health services are considered. Services were initiated on the basis of a somewhat limited medical model. The greater recognition of psychiatric disturbance led to an expansion, perhaps an over-expansion, of the medical model in attempts to provide services for psychologically disturbed students. Contributions came from medicine, psychiatry, psycho-analysis, education, educational psychology, psychometrics and counselling. It is not surprising, therefore, that theoretical concepts are confused and methods of treatment often pragmatic. There are cogent reasons for attempting clarifica-tion at the present time. Medical and counselling services at universities are going through a phase of reappraisal and change and the interrelationships of various methods of giving help are being examined. In the non-university sector of higher education new services are being established, and structures determined now will set patterns for the future. There is a growing recognition in the com-munity of the great lack of services for adolescents and late adolescents with psychological problems. The development of services, their structure and method of operation will inevitably be based on conceptional models involving ideas about 'health' and 'ill health', 'disturbance' and 'normality'.

Methods of case management are derived from these concepts. Fresh problems arise from increasing recognition of the effects on individuals of physical and social aspects of the environment.

I shall describe some of the assumptions and models that lay behind the initia-tion, development and changes in university health services in this country. In the mental health area, further accounts will be found in refs. 1–3. I want to illustrate the importance that models have had in shaping the scope and organization of services and their activities and how, despite their importance, they have received little critical appraisal. Currently, particularly in the area of mental health and the psychotherapies, new explanatory frameworks proliferate and daily add to the repertoire of what may be attempted. Evaluation lags far behind. The state of our current practices in this area may be summarized as one of largely pragmatic methods, with an infrastructure of confused theoretical concepts drawn from medicine, psychiatry, psychoanalysis, education and educational psychology, and counselling. The fact that research has usually been confined within the boundaries of one theoretical framework, despite recognition that the problems cross such boundaries, has contributed to the lack of linkage between clinical and research efforts.

I shall now survey some aspects of the way in which services have developed. A fuller account is provided by Mair.[4] After the Boer War much concern was expressed at the deplorably low standard of physical health of recruits, and this concern eventually led, after various commissions and enquiries, to the establishment of the School Health Service. Some years later, questions were asked about the responsibilities of *university* authorities for the welfare of their students. Two models were implicit then in the thinking. Health was defined in physical terms and located in a physical illness–fitness dimension within the individual. Problems of psychological wellbeing were thought of as lying within a moral spiritual framework, one properly and exclusively the concern of educators or spiritual advisors. Thus the limited activities which were then initiated took the form of attempts to identify individual physical defects and to promote something termed health by physical exercise and gymnastics with the aid of part-time physicians and physical education instructors. Little more than this was attempted until well into the 1940s, when several reports appeared, endorsing this type of approach and recommending that student health departments should come under the general direction of Departments of Social and Preventive Medicine. The environment was acknowledged as being important for physical health, but the universities took comfort from the fact that they were not within any stringent legislative framework, so that most activities in this area were desultory and piecemeal.

With the introduction of the National Health Service in 1948 debate began about whether university services should continue to have a role solely of prevention and early detection without any therapeutic responsibilities (on an industrial health model) or whether facilities for treatment should be included. There was considerable discussion and dissent at this time amongst university physicians.

In the early 1950s, psychiatry burst upon the scene with the publication of Parnell's paper[5] on *psychiatric* morbidity and suicide. The interest and alarm generated had several effects, including the enlarging of the medical model to include states of psychiatric disturbance. As more states of disturbance began to be recognized we entered an era of psychiatric nosology, during which workers sought to delineate, identify, count and generally comprehend the somewhat bewildering diversity of syndromes. There was a search for methods of classification, hope for comparative studies, and hopes for aetiological understanding. Though most of these hopes were unfulfilled, undoubtedly much was clarified in these years and, at the same time, interest shifted from the limited role of detection and prevention to a much wider responsibility including the provision of therapeutic resources. Also, at the same time, there was a general trend for services to be integrated with the National Health Service and to establish general practice lists, which provided a setting in which more and more problems declared themselves.

Changes continued to take place in psychiatric thinking. In some universities, at least, the impact was felt of the Princeton Conference of 1956[6] (chaired by Erik Erikson). Psychological models dealing with growth and development, intrapsychic conflict and concepts such as identity extended interest from nosology into a framework of psychodynamics. One result was the stimulation of attempts to set up psychotherapeutic recourses as part of what a university might provide—the focus of such therapy being an intrapsychic change. The costs of implementing this in any substantial way would have been formidable.

The focus of the various models so far has been the student as an individual —but the social sciences have not been without influence and have reminded us of the important ways social forces act in society and in an institution. Those who place maximum emphasis on what they term the sick society may even oppose the establishment of services that help the individual, on the grounds that this was a device for shoring-up a collapsing social framework and, therefore, detrimental in that it hindered radical change. The diversity of frameworks provides plenty of scope for confusion when several individuals confront the same problem. The student who does not work, for example, sees his problem as caused by the defects and inadequacies of his course. His tutor refers him to the university health service with a hope that his inability to work may be due to physical or psychological ill health. The physician or psychiatrist finds no definable physical or mental disturbance and re-defines the problem as motivational, so returning it from the clinical frame of reference to an educational one. One beneficial effect of the social sciences has been that they have obliged us to think in interactive terms and to take account of the interplay between forces within the individual and forces within his context.

Into this situation with its complexities and confusions we now have to welcome a new developing group of professionals—the counsellors, with models and methods of their own. Disturbance is not always illness; patients become clients, and therapists counsellors. In the most highly developed services the counsellors hope to act as catalysts to the staff—discussing in the community problems and issues as they arise and so, they hope, influencing some of the social forces.

Back in the medical model again, the physical environment has taken on new and important aspects and has become something universities are having to take seriously; the growth of technical and biological research has made laboratories more dangerous than before; at the same time safety and health in universities is now covered by the Health and Safety at Work etc. Act, so that new measures are now required by law. New organizational structures are being developed so that needs can be defined and actions taken to satisfy them. Such activities will have psychological repercussions in the organization. One can already see familiar and not unexpected phenomena developing: for example, denial of hazards, paranoia about bureaucracy, search for a scapegoat when some danger is discovered that needs a lot of scarce resources to put it right. At an individual level, stresses may be generated when change comes at an unfortunate time; for example for those people with research grants sufficient for equipment but not for its safe use. These last points illustrate how the social and organizational environment and the physical environment are closely interacting in practice, as Sergean[7] has emphasized.

I hope I have given some idea of how university health services have changed. I may summarize our present position as the familiar one of new and different demands with static or shrinking resources, and in the next few years we shall have to face some difficult questions. Where do our priorities lie? At present we try to integrate preventive measures and primary care, with a psychiatric and psychotherapeutic back-up, and we are trying to add occupational health. Will all this continue to be viable? With regard to mental health, on what range of models should we base our therapies, and should most of these become non-medical activities? Should some of us attempt to become social pathologists? We can be sure of only one thing. Change will continue and, as Dr Abercrombie reminded us, it will be uncomfortable.

Discussion

Guz: Who funds this service?

Lucas: It is partly funded by the University but some money comes from the National Health Service because some staff members are general practitioners.

Bickerton: Where do the referrals come from?

Lucas: Most students refer themselves. We work in close liaison with tutors and other members of the university staff who, occasionally, initiate referrals.

Bickerton: Nurse management and nursing associations are currently investigating families who do not register with general practitioners. Are the students who commit suicide those who do not accept the service? How do we reach them?

Lucas: This is a central problem. The fact that many troubled students do not avail themselves of the health service was one reason for setting up a university counselling service outside the health service, so that people who feel themselves to be disturbed but do not want to define themselves as ill may know that there is a place where they can seek discussion, without becoming 'patients'.

Guz: How do you exercise your role as a 'factory' health inspector, particularly when, say, faced with a rebellious professor who does not want to know?

Lucas: I don't. The college has set up a safety committee consisting of academic and other staff under an academic chairman with a full-time safety officer. Each department also has its own safety officers. We have recognized the need for more professional advice by appointing a part-time consultant in occupational health.

Knox: It is a striking anachronism that while students in universities and colleges have for some years had available to them the services of qualified counsellors and psychiatrists, students nurses are not provided with this kind of help. Usually the nurse is young, may be living away from home for the first time, and is suddenly confronted with extreme changes in style of living. More often than not she will have to come to terms with death and dying on a terminal cancer ward or in casualty. Is it still assumed, as some nursing tutors have suggested, that all this is a part of character-building, or should we be pressing for counselling services as a matter of course for student nurses, student doctors and trainee ancillary workers?

Lucas: Some other university health services have links with medical schools and hospitals; the health care of nurses forms part of their range of activities.

Knox: I still find it difficult to understand why the *university* health services look after students working in the National Health Service rather than the other way round!

Tait: It is not so strange; think how difficult it is for a nurse or a doctor to be ill. Trainee nurses and medical students build an identity for themselves as givers not receivers of care. To surrender that identity and declare oneself a patient is difficult for many medical students, as it often is for doctors.

Lucas: But it is much easier to declare oneself a patient with, say, appendicitis than to declare oneself as being anxious, troubled, depressed and generally not able to cope. The latter is especially difficult if one has to admit it to a member of the judging part of the profession who may be responsible for assessing one for a house job in a year's time, for example.

Bridger: Although these comparisons are clear, it is essential to distinguish

between the two sets of cases, between those for whom seeking help from counsellors or psychotherapists is still socially acceptable and those who are in a
much more threatened position when seeking such support from someone who
has the power to affect a career or future development.

Russell: As a tutor, I find it difficult with medical students to judge when a
problem has got to the stage when alarm bells should start ringing and someone
else should be consulted. Would it be better for tutors of groups like medical
students, who may be somewhat inhibited about approaching counselling or
other services, to have or to acquire more counselling skills than for yet another
group to be created to whom students could go?

Roy: This is the old problem of formalization. We enquire into interactions,
we think we understand what is going on, but we then feel that we must formalize this knowledge in order to give advice. Maybe we should not give
advice but merely talk to these people; all we can do is lead troubled students
and troubled members of the community to their own solutions. We must be
careful of unduly formalizing counselling services.

Bridger: And before that, perhaps, we should provide the climate and sanc-
tioned means by which people may feel that there is a readiness to receive them
and to discuss or explore their difficulties. On a related theme and returning
again to Dr Abercrombie's paper,[8] is it not more than a possibility that finding
out and understanding things that are happening to oneself is an active intro-
spection leading to insight and a greater capacity for empathy—and even to
doing something about what one perceives?

Abercrombie: What impressed me most when I was working with preclinical students was the stress of being a medical student, especially the sacrilege
of tampering with the dead. Students used to try to overcome this fear in
various nonchalant or jokey ways, referring to the corpse as 'old Harry'. For
example, I was intrigued by the way in which their attitude to dissection affected
their way of thinking about a word such as 'normal'—in discussing the 'normal
body' during the teaching of anatomy, they automatically excluded 'old Harry'
because he had been 90 years old and did not matter (as though an abnormal
person would be likely to survive so long!). Several interesting changes were
then being made in the medical curriculum, and when I told a group of deans
of medical schools at a conference on education about my worry, I received a
frosty response: they had suffered no adverse effects from dissecting. But one
recalled how an eminent surgeon who had seemingly gone through all this
without trauma had told him that whenever he had a nightmare it was about
the dissecting room. For other students the impact comes at their first post-
mortem. We should recognize that these are sources of stress.

McClymont: Dr Lucas, is the counselling service closely identified with the university health service and, with regard to the social acceptability of presenting oneself for help, to what extent are students able to see a link between the two services? Can they perceive the dimensions of health as embracing psychosocial problems?

Lucas: The relationship varies from university to university. At University College, we are in the process of change because a new counsellor is being appointed, but the intention is still to provide a separate mode of entry to a helping service while we maintain professional links between the services. We are anxious to avoid what has happened in some services in the USA, namely, separation into physical health services, mental health services, environmental services and counselling services often with great rivalry and lack of collaboration. So far we have been able to resist the increasing pressures for fragmentation.

Huntingford: Why are medical students not generally provided with the kinds of health services you described? Why do doctors in particular find it difficult to take time off when ill? The answers may be connected with the use of the word counselling, which implies talking rather than listening. Many people do not derive satisfaction from consulting doctors, because their voices are not heard and because the doctors feel compelled to talk. One of the radical changes that is required in medicine is to make it fit people. Doctors feel that they have to do something, and are unable to accept the principle that listening is a positive action sufficient in itself.

Roy: Therapeutic listening is, more precisely, the avoidance of the temptation to be constantly giving advice.

Goulston: This art of listening is something that in general practice we are developing more and more. After 20 odd years I am beginning to learn to listen. Some people think they listen but fail to understand the real meaning behind the words. In this, I accuse medical colleagues other than general practitioners, because, happily, modern general practice is concentrating on this aspect of the interview. Listening is one of the most difficult arts; to learn not to talk too much in one's consultation (an objective I am coming to as a gut reaction) is fundamental to the type of medicine in which I am involved.

Roy: An explanation for the inability to listen may lie in traditional clinical teaching: the hospital consultant usually teaches students how to take histories. If the patient continues for more than two sentences, the student is then instructed to stop the patient because the system for taking histories has been formalized and the student must follow that formality. I have been encouraging my students to let the patient talk for five or even ten minutes and to formalize the conversation later.

Bridger: Apart from emotional reasons, difficulty in listening can be attributed to, first, an increase in the use of the computer or other procedures which need selected information to be processed in certain forms and, secondly, to an educational system in which talking, speaking and writing are emphasized but listening is not.

Tait: We teach a medical student a restricted form of medical history taking. He is taught to ask questions rather than listen. If he is to be able to deal with the emotional and social problems presented by his patients he must be taught to listen, and to ask questions in a different way.

Knox: Curiously, many of the problems of today have arisen, been understood and, sometimes, dealt with in history. Hippocrates taught his pupils to observe patients holistically—to take into account their life-style and their environment by going to the market place and listening to the 'noise of the people'. In the 16th century, Vesalius, writing of the decline of medical practice during the Middle Ages in his *De Fabrica Humani Corporis*,[9] castigated doctors who 'despising the work of the hand began to delegate to slaves the manual attentions they judged needful for their patients and themselves merely to stand over them like architects', and who 'declined the unpleasant duties of their profession without however abating any of their claim to money or to honour'. More recently, Pulvertaft[10] proclaimed the 'heresy' that medicine can never become fully scientific unless it becomes completely inhuman. Dr Roy's students may be encouraged to emulate the advice of one of the founders of their profession and resist the further dehumanizing of the transaction between themselves and their patients.

Joyson: This is the first time for many years that I have heard medical staff indicating that they have time to listen. Their inability to give time to listen to patients has always been a great problem. However, I am concerned that individual counselling causes dependence rather than acts as an encouragement to independence. I strongly support the idea of occupational health services within hospitals as I feel we should care as much for each other as we do for our patients. Listening to each other is an integral part of the service. I agree with Dr Abercrombie that group sessions should be used much more to create this self-supportive atmosphere within a hospital.

McClymont: We have noticed that nursing students who enter for training as health visitors are frightened initially of the use of silence in a discussion, yet after a short while find it most useful and transforming. They later comment on the tremendous help and revelation that silence has brought in helping them to look more deeply into the problems of patients and clients.

Bickerton: I have recently been dealing with mothers who have had block bookings (i.e. with several other mothers at the same session) at paediatric departments. These mothers are not listened to; the paediatrician does not have time to listen and the mothers know that they cannot talk after they have been sitting for a long time with a screaming child in an outpatient department. In one maternity hospital, for instance, the smallest baby ever born there survived and eventually was discharged, care of the mother. Each time she came back to outpatients, everybody gloated over this baby and praised its progress but ignored the mother's complaints about the child's crying. Finally, the mother killed the baby. The reaction at the hospital was 'how dare she kill *our* baby'. This exemplifies the need to listen and to give the mothers the opportunity to talk.

Knox: There is the obverse of listening—for instance, the woman who is counselled in hospital on how to feed her baby. It seems that, increasingly, nurses who teach breast-feeding are not, on the whole, women who breast-feed their own babies and consequently there is a direction towards not breast-feeding. Attitudes can become twisted around; a recommendation by a knowledgeable person, for example, a nurse, can be passed on to the patient.

Bridger: Many of these comments also lead towards the significant work of Isabel Menzies[11] in her study of nursing in a hospital. She showed how frequently the organizational structure could not only be designed or used for the purpose of achieving the objectives of the institution but also for the purpose of defending the people in the system from various anxieties in their work and relationships. Our listening can be used similarly, consciously or unconsciously, for relevant purposes or to defend ourselves against certain anxieties.

References

[1] LUCAS, C.J. & LINKEN, A. (1970) Student mental health; a survey of developments in the United Kingdom, in *University Mental Health* (Pearlman, S., ed.), Brooklyn College of the City University, New York

[2] LUCAS, C.J. & CROWN, S. (1974) Concepts and methods in student mental health. *British Journal of Psychiatry 125*, 595–603

[3] PAYNE, J. (1969) *Research in Student Mental Health*, Monograph, Society for Research in Higher Education, London

[4] MAIR, A. (1967) *Student Health Services in Great Britain and Northern Ireland*, Pergamon Press, London

[5] PARNELL, R.W. (1951) Mortality and prolonged illness among Oxford undergraduates. *Lancet 1*, 731–733

[6] FUNKENSTEIN, D.H. (ed.) (1956) The student and mental health on international view (Proceedings of the First International Conference on Student Mental Health, Princeton, New Jersey), Riverside Press, Cambridge, Massachusetts

[7] SERGEAN, R. (1973) in *Occupational Health Practice* (Schilling, R.S.F., ed.), Butterworth, London

[8] ABERCROMBIE, M.L.J. (1976) The difficulties of changing, in *This volume*, pp. 3–11

[9] VESALIUS, A. (1543) Preface to *De Fabrica Humani Corporis fabrica libri semptem*, Basel

[10] PULVERTAFT, R.J.V. (1952) The individual and the group in modern medicine. *Lancet 2*, 839–842

[11] MENZIES, I. (1960) *The Functioning of Social Systems as a Defence against Anxiety*, Tavistock Pamphlet No. 3, Tavistock Institute, London

General discussion I

The medical profession, patients and society

Huntingford: In her paper,[1] Dr Abercrombie seemed to say that change was intolerable beyond a certain point and, therefore, might produce undesirable effects. I like to feel that change can go as far as it will and result in nothing but good in the long run. Furthermore, I must question the assumption that has been running through the discussion so far that we need organized health care.

Dr Abercrombie referred to Escher's painting illustrating egocentricity and said that by working in a group we can enlarge our own egocentric views. Is the medical profession a group and, if so, does it have a wider view than the individuals who compose it do? I am unable to accept that the medical profession is a group in this sense. In which case, what does the medical profession represent? In my opinion the biggest single problem that we face in providing health services is the attitudes of the profession. But before we can influence these attitudes we need to know what the profession is in Dr Abercrombie's terms.

Roy: Bernard Shaw said that 'a profession is a conspiracy against the laity'. We must acknowledge the truth in this statement and the implied rebuke.

Tait: Medicine can in a sense be seen as the model for the way a profession behaves in relation to society as a whole. Looking at the history of medicine we see that, first, an area of special expertise is defined, then a body of knowledge and skills is built up and restricted to the professional group through control of the educational process. Finally, the exercise of the skills of the profession is denied to anyone outside by law. This may be seen as a protection of public interests but it also places the profession in a powerful position of monopoly, which can be abused. The services of medicine now seem to be so important to society that it will no longer tolerate the delivery of medical care being left primarily in the hands of the profession. In this new situation medicine has once again to lead the way and to discover how to satisfy the conflicting demands of society and a profession.

Arie: We must not forget the external forces that society applies to the medical profession to shape its pattern of practice. At a previous Ciba Foundation symposium,[2] this was a central topic of discussion with Ivan Illich, whose thesis is that medicine expropriates health from people.[3] However, society may also expropriate judgement from medicine. What the public insists that a doctor should do for them is not always what doctors want to do; society finds it convenient to maintain the uniqueness of the doctor and this makes the substitution of other personnel for doctors more difficult, because the public insists that certain things may be done only by doctors. Some things are not appropriated by, but assigned to, the medical profession; for example, the legitimization of the sick role in circumstances of doubt, when it is often not sapiential knowledge on the doctor's part that is required but rather that the doctor should legitimize what is often no more than a self-assessment by the patient. In other words, some of the closed shop of medicine is demanded by the public. Many other factors apply, too, but we should not lose sight of this.

Human beings seem to have a curious propensity to polarize issues and to take up a position at one or other pole—for many reasons, in part to do with personality or sometimes through having spent too much time at the other pole. Take Dr Birley's provocative analogy of the pyramid with arrowheads pointing up or down (p. 29). We know (and he knows) that solutions are not often as easy as he proposes; there *are* important reasons why the person with the overview tends to be more highly valued than the person who has a view of detail only. There are equally strong reasons why sometimes the emphasis should be on the latter. This is the old argument about whether in an army the private or the general is more important. The answers to such questions are not likely to be found at one pole or the other; they are balances. We have to balance many factors before we take up positions on such matters. For instance, it is commonly held that the doctor's only concern should be the interest of his patient. Except in societies in which medicine is an elitist activity denied to the mass of the people, this can hardly ever be so, because any decision to do something for one patient is also a decision not to do something for other people—a disbursal of finite resources (e.g. a hospital bed or regular psychotherapy) to one person means that it is no longer available to other people who have, or might have, a claim on it. This attitude, incidentally, is reinforced by the reorganization of the National Health Service in the sense that medicine is now reorganized on a district basis; doctors now know who are the people who might have a claim on their service and should be better able to balance the demands of an individual against the potential demands of a defined group. The individual and the group represent not polarities but balances. Other examples of polarities are the respective importance of the periphery and the centre; how much should be done by the specialist team in the hospital and how much by the primary care unit; the human and the technological; and acute and chronic care in the health service. Yet we cannot simply provide care for common conditions and altogether ignore the complicated ones. Then, do we need more data or more ideas? All these things must be resolved as balances, and not as polarities.

Roy: Why is it that intelligent people when they become patients suspend their normal power of judgement? We have all listened to friends relating their experiences in hospital or private consulting rooms where, apparently, the most bizarre conversations have taken place and they have accepted without question advice that was obviously unsound. These people, who would question their lawyer or accountant most carefully, erect a barrier to logic when confronted with a doctor. If we are talking about making health care the responsibility of ordinary people, we must teach them to exercise their judgement on these matters.

Beckhard: The professions have been studied[4] in a variety of perspectives, including power. One definition of power (maybe not the common one) is the capacity to control others' destiny, by the use of rewards and punishments, as seen by the people, groups or organizations on the receiving end. Power is always relational and perceptual; parents do not have power over children but children give it to them, in different amounts at different ages. If we accept this definition and tie it in with Dr Roy's comment, we see that the patient, because of his or her need for protection against anxiety, gives the doctor power, whether the doctor wants it or not. Frequently, the doctor colludes in this act. We want those patients to be less dependent and to take more responsibility on themselves—we wish that they would, in effect, grow up. I suggest that doctors and other health professionals have to recognize the normalcy of this attribution of power and consequently have to alter their own behaviour if they want to wean the patient from total dependence.

Huntingford: We have to break this collusion between the profession and those we serve if we are to change the power relationship. Such change will be painful for the profession and individuals, because removal of power implies rejection of doctors. If one can accept such change without being hurt (or if one enjoys being hurt), no harm is done to the profession. But in any case we must break down the barriers that polarize issues and attitudes. Rather than teach people doctors should learn from them. If people are not willing to accept independence from me as a doctor, I feel that I should reject what they ask of me.

Beckhard: If the doctor and the patient were to agree and understand that the task on which they were both engaged was improving the patient's health, the condition would differ from that which usually exists—i.e. the patient considers that it is the doctor's job to get him well and the doctor considers that it is the patient's job to get well. The power differential centres on the maintenance of this difference. I suggest that the doctor, who is perceived as powerful, can help the patient to focus on the common task.

Bridger: In other words, shared collaboration rather than either/or.

References

[1] ABERCROMBIE, M.L.J. (1976) The difficulties of changing, in *This volume*, pp. 3–11
[2] ILLICH, I. (1975) The industrialization of health, in *Health and Industrial Growth (Ciba Found. Symp. 32)*, pp. 157–169, Elsevier, Excerpta Medica, North-Holland, Amsterdam
[3] ILLICH, I. (1974) *Medical Nemesis: the expropriation of health*, Calder & Boyars, London
[4] CARNEGIE COMMISSION ON HIGHER EDUCATION (1972) *Professional Education: Some New Directions* (Schein, E., ed.), McGraw-Hill, New York

Implications of shortening the time spent in hospital

C. J. ROBERTS

Department of Community Medicine, Welsh National School of Medicine, Cardiff

Abstract The decision to shorten the time spent in most areas of hospital care is extremely complex and hinges on the balance of numerous resulting credits and debits, which are largely unknown. The length of stay in hospital can be stabilized for many categories of medical care but the likely benefits may be disappointingly small in the face of unchanged demand for health care. Furthermore, a sustained reduction in length of stay could bring with it logistic, contractual and personal problems, the costs of which could outweigh the benefits of stabilization. The best delivery of health care in a closed financial system seems to depend on a joint consideration of output per unit time and a provision of a service that comes near to satisfying the true need for that service. The appropriate level of service will be decided from a study of the true prevalence of the need and the ability of the service to satisfy it. The enthusiastic pursuit of traditional efficiency without adequate information may be counterproductive—by increasing demand, by demoralizing the health personnel and by diverting some of the demand into private practice. Our first priority is the rationalization of demand; this will need the combined efforts and goodwill of the consumer and the supplier. Only when demand has been rationalized may we expect a net benefit from shortening length of stay.

Between 1949 and 1961 the volume of work done in hospitals in the UK steadily increased; the number of new outpatients examined annually rose from 6.2 to 7.2 million and the number of inpatients from 2.9 to 4.3 million—a rise of 48%. In contrast, the average number of occupied beds rose until 1954 but fell thereafter because the average stay of an inpatient was continually shortened from over 49 days in 1949 to 34 days in 1961. By 1972 the average stay for all causes (except maternity and psychiatric diseases, including mental handicap, requiring patients to be kept in hospitals for the treatment of such diseases) had fallen to 16 days.[1] This decline is partly due to improved methods of treatment; to earlier discharge, particularly after surgery; to changes in the policy of admitting patients to hospital; and to the rising number of patients admitted briefly for diagnostic tests rather than treatment. Had the average length of stay in hospital not declined it would have been necessary to embark upon a major expansion programme if hospitals were to provide the service expected of them. The shortening length of stay has been a prominent feature of hospital care since the inception of the National Health Service, but it may be salutary to consider whether, more than 25 years on, there is room for further action of this kind.

TABLE 1
Regional variation in length of stay for, and frequency per 100 000 population of, selected operations in England and Wales

Region	Operation							
	Thyroidectomy		Division and ligation of oviducts		Removal of tonsils and adenoids		All operations	
	l.o.s.[a]	o.r.[b]	l.o.s.	o.r.	l.o.s.	o.r.	l.o.s.	o.r.
Newcastle	9	19	8	128	4	262	9	5602
Leeds	9	15	9	58	3	299	10	5809
Sheffield	7	18	10	56	4	205	9	4754
East Anglia	15	22	10	39	3	255	9	4833
N.W. Metropolitan	10	20	11	37	5	304	10	5961
N.E. Metropolitan	10	31	10	39	5	317	10	6168
S.E. Metropolitan	10	26	9	36	5	329	10	5925
S.W. Metropolitan	11	26	11	29	5	333	10	6241
Wessex	8	22	11	27	4	385	9	5952
Oxford	9	18	8	38	3	399	7	6090
South Western	10	19	8	68	4	300	9	5599
Wales	11	32	9	62	4	280	10	5977
Birmingham	26	24	9	31	4	250	9	5297
Manchester	10	23	9	89	3	362	10	6130
Liverpool	10	17	9	133	4	251	10	5442

[a] Mean length of stay.
[b] Number of operations per 100 000 population; figures to the nearest whole number.

Table 1 shows the regional variation in length of stay of patients after selected operations in England and Wales in 1972.[1] The operations were selected not because of a prior suspicion that the consequent length of stay varied substantially in different hospitals but because they were well defined and standardized procedures in common use. The greatest variation was found in thyroidectomy and the least in the removal of tonsils and adenoids. For thyroidectomy the average time spent in hospital was 26 days in the Birmingham region compared with seven days in the Sheffield region. The methods of the surgeon, demand for beds, and perhaps even some differences between patients are among the more obvious reasons for such variations, but if patients discharged after seven days were fit, why keep them in for 26? Conversely, if a longer stay were beneficial why were some patients discharged too soon? As inpatient costs in a district general hospital are now about £20 per day, there would seem to be a good case for shortening the length of stay whenever possible, as long as the patients' health is not prejudiced.

TABLE 2

Regional variation in length of stay in hospital and discharge rate for selected diseases in England and Wales[1]

Region	Disease					
	Congenital dislocation of hip		Acute myocardial infarction		All causes[c]	
	l.o.s.[a]	d.r.[b]	l.o.s.	d.r.	l.o.s.	d.r.
Newcastle	17	7	18	247	13	8840
Leeds	22	10	17	239	15	9015
Sheffield	12	8	15	152	15	7005
East Anglia	20	11	21	168	16	7692
N.W. Metropolitan	18	7	20	191	14	8976
N.E. Metropolitan	15	6	19	211	15	9390
S.E. Metropolitan	25	10	21	220	15	9117
S.W. Metropolitan	17	9	24	183	14	9192
Wessex	27	7	17	161	12	8313
Oxford	14	1	23	149	11	8176
South Western	24	5	19	169	14	8172
Wales	31	7	20	214	13	9624
Birmingham	22	10	15	162	13	7158
Manchester	31	9	17	191	17	8733
Liverpool	19	12	21	197	15	8813

[a] Mean length of stay.
[b] Discharges per 100 000 population; figures to the nearest whole number.
[c] Excluding maternity; psychiatric diseases, including mental handicap, requiring patients to be kept in hospitals for the treatment of such diseases are excluded.

Table 2 shows the regional variation in length of stay of patients with selected diseases in England and Wales for 1972.[1] For congenital dislocation of the hip, a condition of relatively low prevalence, the range was 12–31 days, for acute myocardial infarction 15–24 days, and for all causes (excluding maternity and psychiatric diseases requiring the patients to be kept in hospitals specially for the treatment of such diseases) 11–17 days. Although substantial variation in length of stay exists within categories of care, it is much less when all operations, or all causes, are considered together. The tendency for length of stay to average around 9 and 10 days for all operations and between 13 and 15 days for all causes (except in Oxford and Manchester) is remarkable in view of the substantial demographic, environmental, health and economic differences between many of the regions. In terms of use of resources (bed days per 1000 population), East Anglia with 1230 bed days (length of stay × discharge rate per 1000) is similar to Wales with 1251 bed days. Which region is the more efficient?

A recent study of how 59 consultants in Wales managed appendicitis in 1971[2] showed that the mean length of stay was 8.6 days (range 5.0–11.9 days). Among the 12 Hospital Management Committees in Wales the length of stay ranged from 6.9 to 9.8 days. Because of the large number of patients such differences are statistically significant but this does not necessarily imply that they have any meaning in terms of economics or management. However, if every patient's stay after appendicectomy in England and Wales in 1971 (89 300 cases) could have been shortened by one day, the amount saved would have been about £1.3 million, £80 000 in Wales alone.

Table 3 shows the variation in the time women spent in hospital for division and ligation of the oviducts for sterilization, based on all such operations undertaken in Wales in 1973. The range observed is much greater than for

TABLE 3
Variation in time spent in hospital by patients for division and ligation of oviducts in Wales (Evans, P.J., Holgate, S.K. & Roberts, C.J., unpublished data, 1973)

Duration of stay (days)	Number of operations
0	7
1	26
2	118
3	164
4	60
5	91
6	149
7	119
8	155
9	206
10	162
11	112
12	46
13	21
14	19
15–20	21
21+	11
	1487

Mean duration of stay was 7.3 days.

appendicectomy: 4.3–9.1 days between Area Health Authorities and 2.9–11.5 days between hospitals. Consultants working in the same hospital tended to prescribe similar lengths of stay. Table 3 shows two peaks: one at three days and one at nine days. If all Area Health Authorities in Wales adopted the three-day policy some 350 bed days per 100 000 population per annum would be saved and thus beds would be released for further cases of sterilization or other purposes. This would represent a saving of 0.6% of the total annual use of beds for all operations in Wales (i.e. 10×5977 bed days per 100 000 population; see Table 1). The problem is to decide whether the benefits of a 0.6% saving in resources exceed (by an acceptable amount) the costs of implementing such a policy. (A note of caution—there are at present 10 different ways in which female sterilization can be coded and consequently there is considerable opportunity for coding error. Before inferences can be drawn from marginal differences in the Hospital Activity Analysis, there must be good grounds for believing that the data are accurate.)

DISCUSSION OF FINDINGS

During the past 25 years in England and Wales workloads in hospitals have been managed, without increasing the number of beds, by shortening the length of stay. In theory, this should maximize output per unit cost and hence lower the cost of individual patient care, and (given a constant demand) possibly shorten the time outpatients spent on the waiting list. A shortening of stay from five to three days for the removal of tonsils or adenoids in the South West Metropolitan region should substantially improve the waiting time for tonsillectomy in that region, provided that the shorter waiting list did not encourage referrals which might have been previously deterred by long waiting times. Although there is also evidence of variation in length of stay for other conditions, the benefits of shortening the time spent in hospital are not so obvious—for appendicitis, and possibly acute myocardial infarction, the variation is relatively small, although the prevalence is high, and for ligation and division of oviducts, and congenital dislocation of the hip, the variation is large, but the prevalence is low.

The decision to shorten the length of stay in most areas of hospital care is an extremely complex one that hinges upon the balance of numerous consequent credits and debits, the size and even the nature of which are largely unknown. The following considerations seem to be among the more important. Ideally, it should be ascertained (by appropriate work-study methods) whether extra costs will be incurred. For example, will extra duty payments have to be made? Will laboratory investigations have to be done in the evenings? Will sufficient manpower be available at weekends and holidays? And to what extent will shortening the stay shorten the time between admission and operation, and/or between operation and discharge? Will the ensuing shortening of waiting time lead to an increase in demand because the rationing effect of long waiting times has been removed?

Is the procedure which is under review an effective one—i.e. is there a consensus, supported by the appropriate evidence, that the action in question confers substantial benefit upon the recipient? A premature preoccupation with considerations such as length of stay could deflect, or even inhibit, a proper and timely assessment of effectiveness, and achieve a short-term credit which would be heavily outweighed by a long-term debit.

What are the long-term objectives of shortening the time spent in hospital? What is meant by efficiency in terms of delivery of health care? In the case of removal of tonsils and adenoids, is the practice in the Oxford region more efficient than in the Sheffield region? If length of stay is used as the criterion by which to judge this, the answer must be yes; but if an index of use of resources (e.g. bed days per 100 000 population) is the criterion of efficiency, then Sheffield (with 820 bed days per annum) may be more efficient than Oxford (with 1197 bed days per annum). Oxford's output per unit time exceeds Sheffield's, but (assuming that the need for tonsillectomy is the same in both regions and that the procedure is effective) which region provides a service nearest to the true (as opposed to the expressed) need of the population?

If it is thought that, in certain circumstances, shortening the length of stay will produce substantial savings without prejudicing the treatment of the patient, can such a policy be feasibly instituted and will it be acceptable to those who will principally be engaged in its execution, namely hospital consultants and nursing staff? In Scotland, the length of stay has been surveyed for many years and the results of the findings have been regularly transmitted to those concerned. Evidence shows that, in spite of substantial variation of stay for many clinical procedures, such findings have little influence on patient management. Since the feasibility of shortening the length of stay seems to hinge critically on its acceptance by practising hospital consultants, it is important to give some thought to those factors which may influence its acceptance. Clinicians throughout the country tell of the problems imposed by elderly patients, by shortages of hospital doctors and nurses, and of the effects that longer and perhaps more informal holiday arrangements for all grades of hospital staff are having upon the continuity of patient care. These considerations pose problems for the maintenance of a high annual occupancy of beds. We have little information about how much effort is required from the consultant and his nursing staff to sustain enough vigilance throughout the year to maintain, say, a 20%

shortening of stay. In the absence of payment for each item of service, it may not be at all unreasonable for those responsible for the execution of such a policy to look for some alternative form of inducement for maintaining such a high level of economic vigilance. Such inducement need not be financial but could include: involvement of hospital consultants in discussions about those procedures in which a shortening of stay might be expected to produce substantial savings; preparation of up-to-date information that will demonstrate to the clinician the benefits of his vigilance; an undertaking from management guaranteeing the availability and the continuity of supporting staff; and, finally, possibly some indication that thought will be given to the problem of stabilizing demand.

The best delivery of health care in a closed financial system seems to depend on, at least, a consideration of output per unit time (the traditional management efficiency criterion) and the provision of a realistic level of service determined by the necessity and the effectiveness of the procedure in question. At present we have some information about the former (e.g. length of stay, bed occupancy, waiting time, clinic attendances, etc.) but almost nothing about the latter; yet, as Tables 1 and 2 show, variation in the former is relatively small compared with that between levels of service provided. Perhaps the reluctance of clinicians to accept the exhortations of management to find the optimum length of stay stems from the clinicians' intuitive (and possibly sometimes correct) judgement that the advice from the management will occasionally provide, at best, a marginal net benefit compared with that which would derive from a realistic rationing of consumers and other clinicians' demands. There is an urgent need for candid talks between the consumer and the supplier. Perhaps both could be discouraged from making new and increasing demands on the already overburdened National Health Service and encouraged instead to stabilize demand by working closely to try to decide priorities. If doctors are to be expected to undergo what for most will be a traumatic reorientation, namely, an appraisal of the cost of the treatments they use in the light of consequent savings to the State as well as benefit to the individual patient, then the greatest incentive to them would be some indication that the consumer is prepared to do likewise. Community Health Councils could become the agents of the consumer in this process. One important and early development could be the widescale education of the consumer and the supplier about the costs of, and the known benefits deriving from the most often used contemporary treatments. Until some agreement is reached between representatives of the consumer and the supplier on the priorities in health care, and in the provision of service, much of the enthusiasm for traditional efficiency may have been premature, misplaced or occasionally counterproductive. The only exceptions to this generalization seem to be those procedures for which there is evidence of substantial and continuing inefficiency (e.g. possibly an occupancy of beds of less than 40% per annum), and those which are common, always necessary, and generally regarded as effective (e.g. accident services). For the remainder, increasing the turnover of uncommon procedures can be expected to achieve only marginal net benefits (irrespective of necessity or effectiveness). Increasing the turnover of common procedures of questionable necessity and/or effectiveness will undoubtedly produce real short-term savings but, in the present climate of expectancy of even more health care, this is likely to be more than cancelled out by a subsequent increase in demand.

Discussion

Huntingford: We have never asked the consumers how long they would like to stay in hospital and whether they would like to weigh the costs against the benefits, but we should. Before we ask them these questions, however, we must ask them whether they need what is being offered. Do you agree?

Roberts: Yes.

Huntingford: There should not be any conflict between shortening the stay in hospital and providing time to listen. On the contrary, one has to listen most attentively to shorten the stay effectively. If the time spent in hospital is limited to that required for a technical procedure, it is most important that the person is properly prepared; the doctor should receive their questions and provide information in return.

Arie: You are being less than fair to your own specialty; obstetrics *does* allow the consumer some choice—for instance, early discharge after delivery. Other specialties could learn from this. With regard to the relationship between willingness to listen and length of stay, Revans demonstrated[3] a relationship between the length of stay, not only for particular conditions but as a characteristic of whole hospitals, and the willingness of staff to listen to their subordinates. There can be little doubt that the willingness of staff to listen to patients and the flow of communication from the patient right up the hierarchy (of which in a sense he forms a part) is equally important.

Huntingford: For many investigations and operations the patient has to stay in a specialized environment only for the procedure. Afterwards a modicum of care is all that is required; this could be supplied by other people, such as relatives. Therefore, not only is the issue one of length of stay for a technical procedure, but who is going to care for the patient afterwards.

Bridger: In each case it also emphasizes the necessity of identifying who will bear the cost and for what; additionally, who will benefit and in what ways.

Russell: I agree: it is not just the patient as the consumer who is implicated in this but, in the wider context, the family, the general practitioner and the community services. Whether the reduction in time spent in hospital is planned or not, length of stay is steadily shortening. As the resulting burden inevitably falls on the community services in one form or another, there must be a dialogue not just between the potential patient and the health service but within the health service between the different branches. This element has been missing in the past.

Hockey: Just over five years ago we undertook a small study in which we asked the 'consumer' (the patient) whether he wanted to leave hospital earlier than would normally have been the case.[4, 5] It was an experimental project on early discharge; but, in talking about it we do not always recognize that there is no norm for discharge. Patients may agree to leave 'earlier' because they feel morally bound to do so, knowing, or at least believing, that the health service is overloaded. Bias is, there, likely to be introduced. Moreover, in all the costing of the consequences of early discharge, no account has been taken of the hidden costs to the household, let alone to the community services, or of the loss of earnings incurred by somebody having to stay at home, or of the costs of heating, lighting and laundry and so on. And these items are extremely difficult to cost. Also, early discharge adds a tremendous burden to the hospital in-patient service; not only are the patients no longer available to help the nurse with some routine chores in the ward such as taking the tea round, arranging the flowers and so on, but they are all likely to need the nurse's help. This makes for a greater intensity of nursing care and I doubt whether the necessary additional manpower of nurses in hospitals can be maintained; moreover, a constant and rapid throughput of patients may result in some loss of job satisfaction.

Can we really expect waiting lists to be shortened dramatically with the constant change in consumer expectations? Consider, for example, cosmetic surgery: patients are now operated on who would not have been considered for such an operation a few years ago. As long as we take advantage of advances in medical science and technology, I doubt whether there will be a dramatic cut in, let alone an end to, waiting lists. They will be filled up again by patients with other demands.

Tait: The transition from dependency in hospital with its impressive technology to coping on one's own outside is terribly important; time spent on preparing the patient for it is time well spent. The patients in trouble that I see are those who come out of hospital unexpectedly and too early. They become insecure, depressed, and won't go back to work; the end result is often not an economy at all.

Arie: In discussing length of stay we ought to remember that the need for admission to hospital is itself always only relative, even for the most extreme technological procedures: if you are King George VI and you need a pneumonectomy, you have it done at home. What determines whether anyone is admitted to hospital is a balance of the costs, the profit and loss, of doing the operation elsewhere. As someone who works from a hospital, though by no means only in a hospital, I worry about the fashionable movement of staff into what is called 'the community', and the current philosophy, particularly in psychiatry, by which it can be almost shameful to be found working in, or admitting someone to, a hospital. It is not a case of needing to measure only the cost for the community of early discharge but also the cost to the patient coming into hospital and the staff who remain there, in the form of increasing impoverishment of the hospital. There is no right and wrong in this, merely striking a balance; but the cost must be counted in both directions.

Goulston: An extension of this problem is the stage at which the patient goes back to work. Often patients come to me fully recovered from their operation but, because the consultant has decided they must see him in, say, a month's time it is inconceivable that they should return to work before then. The additional economic loss to the community must be considerable.

Elliott: If the patient feels well and you, as his or her doctor, agree, why cannot the patient decide for himself or herself to go back to work?

Goulston: Because the hospital consultant has instructed him to come back to outpatients in a month's time; such is the social stratification of the nation. This is one of the absurdities we are talking about.

Bridger: The patients can behave like bureaucrats!

Paine: The cost of a patient's stay depends on which part of the hospital the patient is in. Some time ago 'progressive patient care' was much discussed. If patients stay in hospital for the extra few days, as the general practitioners want to do, they could be transferred to a self-help ward, where the cost would be lower. Are we doing enough about this sort of transfer, or about the use of the five-day-week ward, and other similar economic measures?

Secondly, if one wants the professionals to discuss with the public what the public needs and what the public wants, is anyone apart from the psychiatrists interested in profiles of morbidity, such as the Camberwell Register (which documents the demand in that area for psychiatric services)? With such a tool, one can tailor the services to suit the public, taking into account the cost/ benefit implications. Dr Birley, why are there registers of this kind in the psychiatric field only and not for example in other specialties such as surgery, neurology and so on?

Birley: Most registers are based on fairly crude administrative indices and diagnostic categories. These give some epidemiological background information, providing a perspective from which one could focus on to a special study, such as the use of five-day-week wards. When it comes to asking the public what they want or need, I am trying to imagine how I would react if the London Electricity Board asked for my views about putting up the voltage to 350 V—certain matters are beyond my technical competence to judge. Presumably, if one of Dr Huntingford's patients complains of a stomach ache and wants an aspirin, Dr Huntingford might refuse and tell him that he had appendicitis, and not do what the patient wants. What the patient wants must often differ from what the patient needs. We seem to be feeling so guilty that we cannot bring ourselves to say this.

Roberts: But let us suppose that for only one out of every 500 patients routinely X-rayed for backache does the result of the radiograph have any beneficial influence on subsequent management. Clearly, there is a benefit and a cost. Who is to say whether the benefit is worth the cost? In my opinion, it is not the supplier of the service who should make this decision. The supplier should use his skills and expertise to devise means by which the costs and the benefits of the technical procedures with which he is associated can be presented to the consumer in a language that he can understand. It is up to the consumer to decide on the basis of this information whether the difference between the cost and benefit is acceptable to him, and the supplier should abide by such a decision.

Birley: You must also inform him about what you are not going to do instead.

Roberts: Exactly. That amount cannot be spent on something else if it is the intention to use it for radiology. The consumer would understand this.

Levitt: I agree; the only useful way we can involve health care consumers is by giving them information on which they can make decisions. To ask someone who comes into a consulting room whether he even wants to be admitted to hospital, how long he wants to stay there, what kind of treatment regime he wants, etc., is unfair because that person has no way of judging between the options. The first priority is to ensure that the discussion is started on an equal footing. Through the community health councils, consumers can help to evaluate health care programmes over a period of time. I was sad that Mr Paine[6] almost ignored health care planning teams; thay could be an extremely useful force, particularly if authorities would consider using members of community health councils as contributors to the discussions. Progress in the participation of community health council members has so far been slow and the councils must certainly do much more work before they can honestly claim to represent the views of the local community about health care. Work remains to be done on both sides. The councils certainly will become more proficient, but first the professionals who know about the services must provide the community—both the community health councils and individual patients—with as much information as they think they ought to have. Neither group knows what questions to ask but health care planning teams could facilitate progress in this most constructively.

Carter: Dr Roberts asked by how much costs would be reduced if the time spent in hospital was shortened but the question should be, are costs increased? As Dr Roberts said, most of the cost of a patient's stay is incurred in the first few days in hospital when the main part of the treatment occurs; the cost during the remaining part of the stay consists mainly of the hotel cost. Fig. 1 illustrates

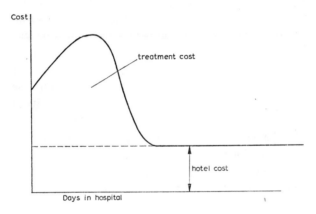

FIG. 1 (Carter). The pattern of incidence of cost during a patient's stay in hospital.

the fluctuation of costs during the patient's stay; this type of curve has been found empirically, for example by Babson.[7] Theoretical models for exploring this have been developed both in Australia[8] and in the UK.[9] In the country as a whole, the average length of stay of a patient has shortened throughout the existence of the National Health Service and is continuing to shorten—to different degrees in different regions although, by and large, the rate of decrease is the same regardless of region. The consequences of shortening hospital stay do not seem to me to be fully realized. If the number of hospital beds and the average occupancy both remain the same, then more patients will be accommodated. This will mean that, overall, hotel costs will be constant but that more treatment costs will be incurred and so the total costs of the hospital service will be increased. What needs to be made particularly clear is that this increase in costs will follow inevitably and necessarily, not as a result of any explicit decision but solely of resources being sucked into the hospital sector. Furthermore, as Miss Hockey pointed out (p. 53) (see also ref. 10), a reduction in the proportion of convalescent patients in a ward will put a further burden of intensive nursing on the nurses and other staff.

Other options are open to us. We could, for example, maintain the occupancy but reduce the number of beds so that the same number of patients could be treated; then costs would be reduced by the capital saving on the beds which have gone. Or, the number of beds could be kept the same but the occupancy reduced until as many patients were being treated as before; the costs would then be reduced but only by the element of hotel cost for each bed-day saved by shorter stay. Intermediate options are also available; these have been explored by Gibbs.[9]

So, a procedure which appears to reduce costs may, and without anyone's conscious decision so to do, *increase* overall costs. It is this aspect of reducing length of stay in hospital that needs particular attention.

Russell: To talk about shortening stay as an end in itself seems to me to be the wrong approach. Is shortening the stay a reasonable way of making limited resources go further? It is not an end in itself; it is what else one can do with the saved time that should be counted as benefit.

Roy: The period between admission to hospital and the institution of appropriate therapy extends the time spent in hospital; this varies considerably and is often overlooked or ignored. It may be used for teaching students but is often an index of inefficiency. Secondly, shortening bed stay may be therapeutically desirable: most of the shortening of the time that patients spend in surgical wards over the last two decades has had little to do with saving money but has resulted from better treatment. As well as the managerial approach to reducing costs by administrative methods, the clinician who shares these aims needs information about how much he is spending on drugs, bed stay and so on in an easily assimilable form before he can make the necessary decisions.

Progressive patient care has not been a complete success; nurses may not like it, especially those in intensive care units who never see the final outcome of their care. Progressive patient care may, therefore, be undesirable because it breaks the continuity of nursing care although it is apparently justified on economic grounds.

Bridger: We have been using the word cost in several different ways—not only in relation to money but metaphorically—for example, to represent the loss of certain current amenities, a cost which a community will have to bear if it also wishes to invest in certain additional services or derive benefit from special innovations and updating of equipment.

Roberts: I tried to question whether it was worth being efficient before demand had been rationalized. Consider tonsillectomy (Table 2): if length of stay is used an an index of efficiency, then Oxford is more efficient than Wales although the annual total use of beds (length of stay multiplied by the operation rate) is virtually the same for both regions (1197 and 1128). But the operation rate for Wales is three per 1000 people compared with four per 1000 in Oxford. If the true need for tonsillectomy is four per 1000 or more then Oxford is undeniably more efficient than Wales; but if the true need is three per 1000 or less, then one per 1000 operations undertaken in Oxford is unnecessary—in which case the net savings from being efficient (in terms of shortening stay) are more than cancelled out by a net loss incurred through unnecessary treatment.

Guz: Dr Carter, what is the cost of not using equipment? Every major hospital has an X-ray department with a vast amount of equipment; it is a prime investigative department and probably the most expensive. No factory manager would dream of switching off 90–99% of his expensive equipment between 5 p.m. and 9 a.m.: that would be considered economic nonsense. Surely somebody can balance the equation of the cost of not using equipment and, say, doing X-ray investigations between 7.30 a.m. and 10 p.m. against the extra cost of staff.

Carter: But what is the cost of not using the equipment? It may be negligible. Are you asking whether more intensive use of the X-ray department enables one to manage, say, with a smaller, cheaper machine, so that one can balance the savings from this against the increased operating cost? If it is not feasible to make this sort of substitution, the question becomes meaningless.

References

[1] DEPARTMENT OF HEALTH AND SOCIAL SECURITY AND OFFICE OF POPULATION STUDIES (1974) in *Report on Hospital In-Patient Enquiry for the year 1972*, HMSO, London

[2] WEST, R.R. & ROBERTS, C.J. (1974) Some observations on the management of appendicitis in Wales. *International Journal of Epidemiology 3*, 351–357

[3] REVANS, R.W. (1964) *Standards for Morale: Cause and Effect in Hospitals*, Oxford University Press (for Nuffield Provincial Hospitals Trust), London

[4] HOCKEY, L. (1970) District nursing sister attached to hospital surgical department. *British Medical Journal 2*, 169–171

[5] HOCKEY, L. (1970) *Cooperation in Patient Care Part I*, Queen's Institute of District Nursing, London

[6] PAINE, L.H.W. (1976) The reorganized National Health Service: theory and reality, in *This volume*, pp. 21–26

[7] BABSON, J.H. (1973) *Disease Costing*, Studies in Social Administration, Manchester University Press, Manchester

[8] DEEBLE, J.S. (1965) An economic analysis of hospital costs. *Medical Care 3*, 138–146

[9] GIBBS, R.J. (1976) Some consequences of the more intensive use of hospital beds, in *Proceedings of Operational Research Society Health and Welfare Study Group Conference* (January 1972), Operational Research Society, London

[10] MOORES, B. (1970) The effect of length of stay on nursing workload. *International Journal of Nursing Studies 7*, 81–89

The nurse's contribution to care

LISBETH HOCKEY

Nursing Research Unit, Department of Nursing Studies, University of Edinburgh

Abstract The concept of health needs as envisaged by the nurse and the challenge of the changing setting to nursing are explored with regard to the nurse's contribution to care against the background of change. Advances in medical science and technology tend to result in increasing specialization in health care and a complex organizational structure for its delivery. These and other factors tend towards fragmentation of care. Care is the concern of all health workers and needs collaboration based on mutual trust and respect.

The nurse makes not the only but a unique contribution to care. In the primary care team she has information about the patient as a 'whole' person and about his or her family on the basis of which she can assess total needs and make appropriate arrangements for these to be met. She communicates with the medical and other members of the health professions in the interest of coordinated and total care, including continuity of care between home and hospital, where appropriate. In hospital, nurses are the only professional workers providing a continuous and direct caring service.

Care is a concept implying a measure of constancy and continuity. These two aspects, reinforced by communication, coordination, explanation, education and empathy, are some of the main components in the nurse's contribution to care.

The emphasis in this symposium is on health needs in a changing setting, but health itself is a subjective value-laden concept, liable to change over time and relative not only to the individual but to the value system of the society. However, within any system of health care, 'the basic need of a sick patient is the need for personal care provided in a way which is conducive to the preservation of his dignity and self respect'.[1] Nobody would dispute that such care is largely the nurse's role and nobody would claim that this role is new. Nursing did not set itself up as a novel discipline—it evolved in response to a need, a need for the care of the sick in body and in mind. Florence Nightingale made the distinction between nursing the sick and nursing sickness; this distinction is becoming more rather than less important. I submit that the nurse's contribution to care in the context of change is her* care of the person, rather than the treatment of a condition.

---

* Although a nurse may be female or male, I shall use the feminine gender in this paper; masculine is reserved for the patient.

Nurses in many parts of the world have for some years attempted to define their activity. At the risk of being branded a heretic by my peer group I am prepared to express my regret that so much time, effort and frustration has been expended in such efforts. I tend to agree with the American nurse, Frances Storlie, who is quoted[2] as having said: '... The glorious thing about nursing is that it cannot be defined, the irony that we never give up trying ...' Notwithstanding my reservations about the worth of defining nursing, it seems appropriate to quote the classic definition produced by the American nurse, Virginia Henderson, which formed the foundation for the International Code of Nursing:[3] 'The unique function of the nurse is to assist the individual, sick or well, in the performance of those activities contributing to health or its recovery (or to a peaceful death) that he would perform unaided if he had the necessary strength, will or knowledge and to do this in such a way as to help him gain independence as rapidly as possible'.

More recently, the Committee on Nursing, under the Chairmanship of Professor Asa Briggs, stated in their report:[4] 'Whether nurses are in hospital or in the community; working as part of a team or alone; whether they are tending the physically sick, the psychiatrically disturbed or the mentally handicapped; whether they are counselling young mothers or elderly people; whether they are nursing neonates or attending the dying, their central role is to ensure the care and comfort of the person being nursed, to maintain oversight and co-ordination of that care and to integrate the whole—both preventive and curative—into an appropriate social context'.

It seems, on the face of it, that the concept of nursing has not changed a great deal, yet, it is abundantly clear that what nurses do has changed and is changing all the time. Indeed, the only constant and certain factor in this age of uncertainty is change itself and it is opportune to focus on the implications and challenges of change to an occupational or professional group whose *basic* terms of reference—the care of the sick (as a simple description of nursing)—remain unaltered.

I shall first identify some of the changes relevant to nursing and highlight a few of the problems they pose. Believing that problems have a positive func tion in showing potential, I shall focus on new opportunities for nursing and conclude on a realistic note on the nurse's actual contribution to care now.

First, the changes and their inherent problems: nursing cannot be practised in a vacuum. It needs a recipient of care, a base of knowledge, other professionals and an organizational framework. Moreover, its ambit or direction is determined by society, expressed in terms of values, priorities and allocation of resources. Changes in all these are obvious.

The recipients of care, the patients, have changed and so have their expectations. Patients who need nursing are older and likely to be more severely ill, disabled or handicapped or they may be immigrants, who may pose problems with communication. It is not for me to suggest reasons for these changes, but clearly some are a direct result of medical and technological progress. Patients who 50 years ago would have died from a birth defect, a severe infection or serious accident, now survive and need care. Antibiotics have stepped in between the old person and his best friend, the fatal pneumonia. Life expectancy has increased markedly, a fact which, linked with the trend towards smaller families, smaller homes and an increase in the number of working women, results in more aged, lonely and vulnerable people, many of whom need care. Patients who are no less ill spend increasingly shorter periods under care; this does not necessarily mean that they need less care.

Patients' expectations are moulded by media which are opening up new areas of knowledge with implicit promises of greater benefits; these benefits are then eagerly demanded by many. Other patients remain submissive and accept any treatment or care with embarrassing gratitude. These patients are extremely demanding in terms of the nurse's integrity; their needs must be deliberately explored and the nurse should encourage more active participation with less restraint. The novelty in this situation is the nurse's awareness of concepts such as patient role, depersonalization, hospital culture.

This leads me on to the second relevant area of change, namely, the knowledge base which provides the foundation for the practice of the art of nursing. More sophisticated systems of nurse education and research findings have increased the nurse's data store, making it incumbent upon her to process and use the data appropriately in her decision-making. For example, we know more about patient anxiety,[5, 6] patient vulnerability,[7] and the advantages of individualized patient care.[8] As the frontiers of knowledge are being pushed out, the potential for improving patient care is increasing. As a nurse has to be a woman (or man) of many parts by virtue of her constant availability, nursing touches many other areas of knowledge, such as medicine, physiotherapy, pastoral care. As a professional, the nurse should update her knowledge all the time, a task which, in view of the volume of new information, is not easy. Although it is splendid to have such a rich supply of new information and knowledge, time and opportunity are needed to acquire, absorb and use it.

As already mentioned, nursing is tangential to several other disciplines and, with increasing knowledge and the resulting specialization, the number of other professionals a nurse encounters in the care of her patients is soaring. It is not only the medical profession which proliferates specialties; the trends permeate other health care fields: physiotherapy, stomatherapy (the care of an opening, e.g. as after a colostomy), psychotherapy are but a few examples. There is, moreover, increasing specialization in technical and other para-medical activities. In a modern hospital one finds technicians who run electro-cardiographs only, others who are responsible for taking blood specimens, yet others whose specialty is testing lung function; there are many more. Dieti-cians, ward house-keepers, ward clerks, ward receptionists are important collea-gues for the nurse, as are nursing auxiliaries, domestic workers and voluntary helpers. They are important not merely because the nurse might have to co-ordinate their activities in the interest of the care of her patients, but also because she might find herself standing in for any one of them. Nurses are still biddable, and more and more people are doing the bidding!

One of the most significant changes relevant to the nurse's contribution to care is the reorganized management structure in which she operates.[9, 10] Organizational changes, known to provoke anxiety, have been almost con-tinuous for the last ten years.[11, 12] The present structure is a giant bureaucracy enshrined in a new nursing hierarchy. Its novelty lies in the nursing representa-tion at every level of the hierarchy, with momentous responsibilities for decision making and budgeting at the apex of the huge pyramid and simple task-orien-tated care at its base. The complexity of the organization necessitates the bureau-cracy, which may frustrate the spirit of the system with its emphasis on easy decision-making and on interdisciplinary collaboration in policy-formulation. Inevitably, the distance between 'shop-floor' need and top level policy-making is lengthening and this separation brings with it an increasing need for greater efforts to communicate. Lines of communication, both horizontal and vertical, must first be clearly identified—not an easy task in view of the increasingly complex network.

Having referred to some of the main changes in patients, knowledge base, professional colleagues and organizational structure, I shall now discuss changes affecting the nurse, her ascribed role and function. In the first place, nurses' full-time working hours have been significantly reduced in the past few years and many nurses work part-time. Part-time nursing is a relatively modern phenomenon, caused by the trend in society for more women to get married.[13, 14] The relatively affluent married nurse can afford labour-saving devices and help in the home and she returns to work for interest or to earn the money to pay for luxury items (or both). The less affluent married nurse needs the additional income although she may also be motivated by interest.

The shorter working week and the increase in part-time nursing result in the need for more individuals to provide any given nursing coverage; this means less time for patient contact by each nurse and the need for more nurses for each patient.

Nurses have, moreover, attempted to gain professional status by laying down a standard of professional preparation, a standard of professional practice, regulations of practice and a code of ethics. Although the principles underlying such developments represent progress and as such are completely desirable, their implementation has in many instances brought its own peculiar problems —problems of job delineation and external constraints to nursing activity. I refer to efforts to identify and ban non-nursing duties whether these are at the lay end of the spectrum (e.g. semi-domestic or orderly duties) or at the opposite end where they impinge upon conventional medical work (i.e. immunization or venepuncture). In my view, rigidity in task prescriptions or task taboos is the greatest enemy of professionalism. A professional nurse should have the freedom and the knowledge to make her own decisions to perform those tasks which she considers to be of benefit to her patients and which are within her area of competence. By the same token, she should be expected to use her judgement on work which is best done by other people, either because of their more appropriate knowledge or because of their easier availability.

Problems should be seen as seed beds for progress rather than as sources of frustration; the mere coping with a problem gives a sense of achievement, a reward which a smooth path would not offer.

The problems that I have outlined are positive challenges to nursing. Retracing my points and starting with the changing patient group composed of the elderly, the very ill, the disabled, the handicapped, the dying, I maintain that it is precisely in the care of these patients that nursing, as an art, can come into its own. For many of these patients, medical treatment has little to offer and the nurse may take over almost completely as the provider of care. There is ample scope for independent research in those areas in an attempt to improve practice. Last month I participated in a National Canadian Conference whose theme was 'Does nursing make a difference?'. In relation to the patient groups I mentioned the answer to this question must be clearly affirmative. Nursing makes *all* the difference. The tragedy is that the nursing of the elderly, the disabled and handicapped tends to carry less prestige value and the care of the dying is often marred by a sense of fear, defeatism or abhorrence. But I hope to see nurses clamouring for the opportunity to care for those patients to whom good nursing makes all the difference and to pursue research as doers or as users with understanding and purpose.

Increasing knowledge and information have the potential of generating the desire for them. The acquisition of knowledge is stimulating and rewarding for its own sake, because it widens horizons and points to new possibilities for thought and progress. Moreover, most nurses are keen to give high quality care and appreciate any help they can get. Knowledge relevant to nursing may come from other disciplines as well as from nursing itself; similarly, such knowledge is likely to be relevant to nurses as well as to other health professionals. One should look forward, therefore, to a much greater pooling of knowledge, not only through the printed word but through formal and informal interdisciplinary contact. Thus, increasing specialization could have an enormous unifying function although, left to develop without a deliberate fusing effort on anyone's part, it is liable to become increasingly divisive. The nurse's contribution to care may lie, at least in part, in the promotion of a functional synthesis of disjointed endeavours. I should like to see a significant upsurge in interdisciplinary education and research which would prepare the ground for the kind of team activity that the complexity of modern patient care demands.

Even the giant bureaucracy of the health service has a potential for good, provided that the people within it do not become stupefied or lose heart. The nurse at the apex of the pyramid has an unprecedented opportunity to influence policy at top level and can thereby contribute to care by appropriate allocation of resources. The nurse in the front line of the profession, who in my view is the nurse involved in direct patient care, has the potential of channelling patient-centred information right to the source of policy making. There is, therefore, a new possibility for a direct link between the needs of the patient as perceived by the nurse who cares for him and policy which can facilitate patient-centred care. The novelty in this situation lies in the level of policy making. Before the reorganization of the health service, the limit of the impact of a nurse's decision-making was nursing in a hospital or in a group of hospitals and, in community care, nursing in a small circumscribed area. Now, one nurse in top administration has an influence over the full range of health services both in hospital and in the community. In consultation with other members of the executive team she wields significant power in the shaping of health care provisions, not merely of nursing services. She competes for resources alongside other health professions and it is therefore particularly important for her to be provided with relevant information on which to make her case. Even at this level Florence Nightingale's distinction between nursing the sick person and nursing the sickness may be applicable. The cure of a disease tends to make greater financial demands than the care of an elderly person—it also tends to be more dramatic and to gain ready public approval. The important contribution of the nurse–administrator to care in the changing health care setting is, therefore, the acquisition of resources for care and their appropriate allocation.

This brings me to the nurse's present contribution to care, the use of resources in the interests of patient care. Examples, describing existing but relatively new care patterns and nursing–research contributions to care, are intended to illustrate some general points.

In spite of the integrated health service, to whose philosophy most people would readily subscribe, it is necessary to make some distinctions between hospital and domiciliary nursing.

Hospital nursing presents a challenge to nursing care for the reasons I have mentioned. Nurses are the only professional workers providing a 24-hour caring service for seven days a week. Care is a concept implying a measure of constancy and continuity. Yet the turnover of patients and the turnover of nursing staff, especially in acute wards, militate against the establishment of relationships between individuals and against continuity of care. Task assignment in the delivery of nursing care further complicates the nursing of the patient as a person. Nurses have attempted and are attempting to overcome these problems by evolving team nursing and patient assignment.[15] Such systems vary in detail but the principle lies in the accountability of one nurse or a small team of nurses for the total care of one patient or a group of patients. It is, therefore, easier for individual patient's needs to be identified and acted upon. Patients can relate more easily to a nurse identified as their nurse or a member of their nursing team.

Another innovation in aiding continuity of care is the use of the nursing consultant, who is in some ways analogous to the medical consultant. In such a scheme each patient is, on admission, allocated to a senior nurse with expertise relevant to his condition; she is available for consultation throughout his stay in hospital and acts as a link between him and his ward nurses. Unlike the medical consultant, the nurse consultant has no authority to issue care prescriptions or orders; she acts in a solely consultative capacity to both the patient and the nursing staff. Other varieties of nursing consultancy are emerging.

Even within the conventional structure of nursing, the nurse, especially the ward sister or charge nurse, attempts to take responsibility for the patient and his problems even when these do not seem directly related to the pathological condition which necessitated his admission to hospital. Such a total concern is more effectively acted upon where community nursing staff are able to communicate information about the patient and his home conditions to their hospital colleagues. Similarly, continuity of care between hospital and home is facilitated by an adequate and direct communication system between hospital and domiciliary nurses. In many areas such communication has become common practice, particularly since research findings have pinpointed the undesirable effects of breaks in care.[16, 17] In some parts of the country, purpose-designed liaison schemes have been developed, particularly for those patients whose needs for continued after-care in the community are likely to be prolonged; for example, geriatric and psychiatric patients, patients with degenerative conditions or children with long-term care needs such as cystic fibrosis or spina bifida.

Clearly, continuity of care between hospital and community is of benefit not only to the patient and his family but also to the medical staff in hospital and in general practice. Over a long time with the inherent changes in circumstances, the nurse provides an element of constancy, making it easier to observe the patient's reaction to home care. She can alert the hospital to warning signs of the patient's deterioration or family stress.

The other important function of a nurse in hospital is the coordination of the patient's care. I mentioned the ever-increasing number of people who have specialized tasks to perform. There can easily be an excessive number of interruptions to a patient's rest if the specialized activities, all necessary and helpful in themselves, are not coordinated. During a recent observation period of one hour in a hospital ward, no less than 11 different people wanted to give some sort of attention to one patient: two laboratory technicians, a physiotherapist, a dietician, a medical social worker, a medical student, an auxiliary (to take the patient for X-ray), the hospital chaplain, a senior student nurse (to prepare the patient for treatment), a junior student nurse (to obtain a specimen of urine). The 11th person was the ward sister who spent a trying hour in her valiant attempts to protect the patient.

In order to fulfil her coordinating role, the ward sister or whoever assumes a similar responsibility not only must be available but also must appraise the situation constantly to establish care priorities.

A further contribution to care by the nurse is reassurance of the patient whose new environment and apprehension about his condition are bound to make him anxious. No other worker in the hospital who is available round the clock can reasonably expect the patient's confidence. Nursing research has provided new information on post-operative pain and on methods which nurses can use to relieve it.[6] An American nurse showed in an experiment that several undesirable post-operative effects could be significantly reduced by a nurse who spent some time psychologically preparing her patients before operation.[18]

Rehabilitation tends to carry a connotation of physical exercises. It should, however, be regarded in a much wider sense as preparation of the patient for adjustment to whatever his future health status may be—progress or deterioration. Often neither of the two main rehabilitative professions, physiotherapy and occupational therapy, is involved and it is left to the nurse to give whatever rehabilitative care is needed, which may extend to the patient's family as well as the patient himself.

Often the nurse's caring role is educational. In the wake of medical and technological advance follow confusion, fear and bewilderment. New machines, new terms, new treatments need to be explained. Moreover, the pressure on the health service is almost bound to call for increasing education of the public in safe and intelligent self care. Much of this education is undertaken by nurses who have in their patients a captive and receptive audience anxious to learn how to cope in the future.

Many of the opportunities and contributions to care which I have mentioned as being relevant for the nurse in hospital also apply to her counterpart in the domiciliary field. In addition, however, it is pertinent to draw attention to the district nurse's unique opportunity to contribute to care when working in a functional partnership with general practitioners. Her access to patients' records makes it possible for her to keep vulnerable patients under surveillance although their immediate need for nursing care may not be obvious. She may undertake treatment sessions at the surgery and give nursing advice to patients and anxious relatives. By supplying the doctor and other members of the primary care team with information about patients she adds a valuable dimension to the team's joint effort. In a well organized general medical practice or health centre, the members of the team will consult and collaborate with each other and potential disputes over job delineations can be expected to disappear.[19] For example, the district nurse may sometimes be the most appropriate person to give care to the bereaved, at other times it may be the health visitor. In the light of current knowledge on the vulnerability of the bereaved, the provision of such care is most important.

It would be wrong to finish a discussion of the nurse's contribution to care without any mention of mental subnormality. Some would argue that there has been little or no change in that area and that it is, therefore, irrelevant to this symposium with its focus on change. But I should conclude by mentioning current nursing research on the experimental modification of toilet training for severely incontinent patients.[20] Three years ago the nursing staff in a ward of over 30 such patients spent most of their time in tasks related to toilet. Now, almost all the patients have achieved their target behaviour in toilet training and the nursing staff are able to use their time for activities designed to improve the social quality of life for the patients. In times of economic stringency such as these, already under-privileged areas tend to suffer most. The values of society, reflected in the allocation of resources, seem to accord low priority to mental deficiency. It is, perhaps, this work of a young nurse researcher that is making one of the major contributions to care.

Basic to care is empathy; a nurse extends this empathy not only to her patients and their families but also to her medical, paramedical and domestic colleagues.

Without empathy the nurse's contribution to care in the changing setting would not deserve mention.

I have attempted to outline some major problems generated by the changing setting. Viewing problems as a potential for progress I have indicated some possibilities for such progress. The nurse's current contribution to care may be identified as:

Continuity and coordination
Availability and appraisal
Reassurance and rehabilitation
Education and empathy.

Discussion

Goulston: When devolution comes I hope that Miss Hockey can be seconded to London! To me, the biggest step forward in the care of the patient in general practice has come from the close liaison between general practitioner and nursing colleague. Day-to-day personal contact seems to be most important.

Hockey: The paper transaction of attachment does precisely nothing; what is needed is the spirit that goes with it, demonstrated in the attitudes of the doctor, the health visitor and the nurse. Similarly, the piece of paper that made it possible for us to work together by statute in the reorganized health service does not ensure a united service. There must be a will and determination to make it work.

Bridger: The colleague relationship rather than the doctor–handmaiden one is implied.

Birley: We referred earlier to the distinction between treatment and care (p. 15). The Royal College of General Practitioners has recently analysed the sort of patients who make up most of the practitioners' lists.[21] Could the new nurse whose job you described substantially reduce the number of doctors needed?

Hockey: Do you mean that nurses should take over doctors' functions?

Birley: To some extent they should, and it is most encouraging if they are. They have done so in general practice with regard to visiting, screening and so forth. But the implications need to be thought through.

Hockey: A nurse's role is changing all the time. Medical functions tend to become nursing functions. About 20 years ago nurses did not take blood pressures and over 10 years ago they did not take blood samples. However, a nurse should not aspire to being a pseudo-medical person. Her nursing contribution to patient care should be an additional dimension.

Goulston: Are the two professions moving closer together?

Hockey: Yes. It is in the patient's interest that a nurse should undertake certain functions hitherto undertaken by a doctor. For example, a nurse could take blood from a patient provided that she has been taught how to do it safely and that it is part of the patient's nursing care but she should not take blood from, say, 20 patients in a row at a clinic at one session—that is probably the task of a technician.

Guz: Do nurses in this country or do you, representing some nurses in this country, aspire to become the equivalent of the Russian *feldshers* or the Chinese barefoot doctors?

Roy: Or rather, do you agree that nurses should undertake clinical assessment and institute treatment or referral on their own initiative—as nurse practitioners,[22] in fact?

Hockey: A nurse can make a nursing assessment of the condition and report the symptoms to a doctor, but at present, nursing education does not prepare a nurse to make a medical diagnosis, even though it may do in five years' time. A nurse is a superb observer.

Tait: My attached nurse and I may often do the same things, for instance in the care of the dying. One person will suit one patient better than another and is obviously the person to take the blood sample or whatever. Getting the job done is the important thing, not who does what.

Baderman: Miss Hockey is implying more than she will admit. Nurses are, and have been for a long time, making diagnoses and treating patients. Since Florence Nightingale's day the nurse's role has gradually but continually been changing, just as the relationship between the doctors and the nurses has been. It might be self-limiting and inappropriate for us even to attempt to define treatment, because the relationship that treatment implies is perhaps the safest, most flexible and productive way to consider it in this context. The expression 'non-nursing duties' is anathema to me, not because it is unprofessional or smacks of demarcation disputes but because it is unreal. One does what needs to be done in relation to one's training and competence and in relation to the other services that are provided by other professions at the same time. For instance, there is the old argument about whether a nurse in an Accident and Emergency Department who sees a patient with abrasions should send him away or whether she should decide that the lacerations need stitches and put them in. We need guidelines for such matters to be more open-ended and flexible than you appear to be saying.

Hockey: Current legislation and the values that both my own profession and society hold restrict what I say—my personal views might be misinterpreted as official guidelines. When I worked as a rural nurse in a village some years ago patients expected me to be able to make decisions about referral to the doctor, and I did. Then nobody questioned this; these issues are being aired only now.

Bridger: We have already asked whether doctors can be regarded as a group, i.e. as one profession. Now, we have to ask the same question about nurses. It is becoming increasingly difficult to talk about 'the nurse' or 'the doctor' when we may be talking about a group of professions in each case.

Arie: Probably a more helpful approach in the long-term in thinking about substitution for each other and whether nurses should do doctors' work—a question which presupposes that certain things are nurses' work and certain things are doctors' work—is to look at it from the point of view of the needs of the patient. We have to decide who, in the pool of professions and personalities available, is most likely to meet those needs most effectively. I suggest that this depends on four parameters: (1) the sapiential content of the job— generally, the person best fitted to remove a glioma is a neurosurgeon, but the person to stitch up a cut might be one of several professions; (2) the structure in which we function: for instance, nurses traditionally (in hospitals at any rate) work fixed hours and even the most senior nurses go off duty at the end of their shift. Consequently, certain things which may have to be done after the nurse has gone, even if that nurse knows the patient best, have to be done by someone else. (Doctors are moving in the same direction of shiftwork.) Thus, structure might dictate who does what simply by reason of one person being available at a particular time or the fact that the working pattern is such that he or she can make themselves be there; (3) the personality and attitudes of individuals: some things may be done well by one nurse and not by another; some nurses may enjoy technical procedures while others may be more devoted to straightforward caring for patients; (4) the legal setting—this is not immutable, but it sometimes dictates who does what. It might be more fruitful to think in these terms, rather than to ask how far doctors should be doing nurses' jobs and *vice versa.*

Russell: The concept is excellent, but who decides?

Arie: That raises the thorny issue of teamwork and consensus. Ideally, the team tries, with the patient, to decide his or her needs and how to meet these from within its resources. In practice, this is fraught with difficulties. The Government's Working Party on Social Work Support for the Health Service[23] tried to define 'teamwork'. In essence, we said that the responsibilities of members of the team derive not from the prescription of the head of the team but from the needs of the patient; the distribution of responsibilities is negotiated within the team, who recognize that each member may have contributions to make and that the patient has the right to benefit from those contributions. Having tried to define what the patient needs, we negotiate among ourselves how best the team might meet those needs. This process is familiar in psychiatric teams that work well, but less familiar perhaps in others which may have less fluidity between the constituent members. Certainly, there is, alas, a reality gap between the theory and the practice!

Bridger: This theme indicates the growing similarity between the many different types of organization with respect to the development of relevant opportunities for participation, consultation and decision-making. The design of structures, technological and administrative processes to take account of the quality of working life has led to several trial endeavours requiring collaborative working together with close interdependent relationships, for example semi-autonomous group working or the Volvo experiment.

Goulston: I am rather smug at the moment because we have solved these problems of teamwork in our small group working together in the district with real give and take. We form a complete team with superb nurses and excellent health visitors and, soon I hope, we shall have social workers as well. But the complexities of a hospital form a totally different problem.

Baderman: I want to re-emphasize the cultural element. The way in which teams function can be defined in terms of the parameters Dr Arie mentioned, but such a situation seems to me to be a fluid one when considered over a period of time or from one geographical location to another, either within the same country or in neighbouring countries or even from one community to the next. It is an interesting exercise to assess what cultural forces are at work in deciding the various roles that people declare for themselves (so that everybody knows what they are doing, although that itself introduces a certain amount of rigidity while clearing the air—perhaps it is the price one has to pay), what cultural forces induced the current situation, and how they can be moulded and changed to make 'better' use of the resources. (Better is a difficult word here because it carries cultural overtones about what is better.)

Beckhard: Our studies on interdisciplinary health teams over the past five or six years lead us to an alternative definition of a team—a group of people who must be able to pool each other's resources in order to do some task. The tasks define the composition of the team. If one accepts this definition, then the key variable in team effectiveness is not whether the members of the team make decisions consensually or have good communication but whether they all have the same priorities and values about the mission (i.e. patient care) —resources, specialist background etc. We have found that the greatest problem for the team is to agree about that. Once that is agreed other considerations are subsidiary. This agreement leads to a further issue: what contributions do the team members consider they can make to this mission of care, i.e. their role expectations (as opposed to role definitions). This is one way of thinking about how to reallocate these resources if one accepts the above definition of a team. Mutual respect and the desire to collaborate are important but secondary to allocation of resources.

Arie: The two definitions are the same, because the definition I quoted started from the needs of the patient, which determine the roles within the team.

Beckhard: I was distinguishing consensus in decision-making, which is a necessary process, from consensus about purpose, which is the critical condition.

Knox: We keep saying that the consumer has a role to play (vital or not) but when we start to consider the team and the enterprise of care we expel the patient from the team. I wonder how feasible, possible or acceptable it is to allow the patient a function within the context of the health care team.

Hockey: In an interdisciplinary educational system I should like to see a health care college rather than the present pattern where all the different disciplines are educated on a separatist model. At present, nurses are often taught by doctors but the medical student in practice on the ward is taught by the ward sister, who probably instils in him ideas about his medical craft. Most doctors recognize this. If we could all collaborate officially to learn together about patient care we might understand each other, we would have mutual respect and we would appreciate each other's contribution.

Bridger: This is recognized and established in some of the recently founded teaching hospitals, such as Southampton.

Beckhard: The new Institute for Health Team Development in the USA is collaborating with five universities on such an arrangement—interdisciplinary teaching teams of doctors, nurses, dentists, social workers, etc., with some courses cutting across the school of medicine, nursing, dentistry etc. (see ref. 24).

Lucas: We mentioned the importance for the doctor of listening and, with regard to the primary care team, we laid great emphasis on the nurse's listening skill as well as the nurse's problems in combining technical activities that call for a certain amount of busyness with the relaxation that is conducive to the development of listening skills. In the university health service, many people opt to talk to the nurse first; and sometimes she may deal with the matter without referral to the doctor.

Guz: Miss Hockey, do you represent yourself, in which case I have nothing but the greatest admiration for you, or do you represent the nursing hierarchy and their views on the current role of the nurse? I ask because the nurse of the future that you described is so magnificent and so unlike what I see. Even though the nurses in the big hospitals in London are of high academic quality, they are prevented from doing what we think and obviously from what you think they should do by the attitudes of the nursing hierarchy.

Hockey: I am speaking for myself; I have **not** been given a mandate by my professional organization to speak on its behalf. At the moment I cannot be sure that I express the view of the profession as a whole.

References*

1 SCOTTISH HOME AND HEALTH DEPARTMENT (1972) *Nurses in an Integrated Health Service*, p. 1, HMSO, Edinburgh
2 quoted in: CAMPBELL, A.V. (ed.) (1974) *Why Professions*, Contact, New College, Edinburgh
3 HENDERSON, V. (1961) *Basic Principles of Nursing Care*, p. 3, International Council of Nurses, London
4 DEPARTMENT OF HEALTH AND SOCIAL SECURITY AND SCOTTISH HOME AND HEALTH DEPARTMENT (1972) *Report of the Committee on Nursing* (Chairman A. Briggs), Cmnd. 5115, para. 137, HMSO, London
5 MUNDAY, A. (1973) *Physiological Measures of Anxiety in Hospital Patients*, The Study of Nursing Care Research Project, series 2, number 3, Royal College of Nursing and National Council of Nurses of the United Kingdom, London
6 HAYWARD, J. (1975) *Information—A Prescription Against Pain*, The Study of Nursing Care Research Project, series 2, number 5, Royal College of Nursing and National Council of Nurses of the United Kingdom, London
7 STOCKWELL, F. (1972) *The Unpopular Patient*, The Study of Nursing Care Research Project, series 1, number 2, Royal College of Nursing and National Council of Nurses of the United Kingdom, London
8 GRANT, N. (1975) The Nursing Care Plan 2. *Nursing Times*, Occasional papers
9 DEPARTMENT OF HEALTH AND SOCIAL SECURITY (1972) *National Health Service Reorganization: England*, Cmnd. 5055, HMSO, London
10 SCOTTISH HOME HEALTH DEPARTMENT (1972) *Nurses in an Integrated Health Service*, HMSO, Edinburgh
11 MINISTRY OF HEALTH AND SCOTTISH HOME AND HEALTH DEPARTMENT (1966) *Report of the Committee on Senior Nursing Staff Structure* (Chairman B.L. Salmon), HMSO, London
12 DEPARTMENT OF HEALTH AND SOCIAL SECURITY, SCOTTISH HOME AND HEALTH DEPARTMENT AND WELSH OFFICE (1969) *Report of the Working Party on Management Structure in the Local Authority Nursing Services* (Chairman E.L. Mayston), HMSO, London
13 SKEET, M. & RAMSDEN, G.A. (1967) *Marriage and Nursing* (A Survey of Registered and Enrolled Nurses), The Dan Mason Nursing Research Committee of the National Florence Nightingale Memorial Committee of Great Britain and Northern Ireland, London
14 HOCKEY, L. (directed by) (1976) *Women in Nursing*, English University Press, London, in press
15 PEMBREY, S. (1975) From work routines to patient assignment. An experiment in ward organisation. *Nursing Times 71*, 1768–1772
16 HOCKEY, L. (1968) *Care in the Balance—a study of collaboration between hospital and community services*, Queen's Institute of District Nursing, London
17 SKEET, M. (1970) *Home from Hospital*, The Dan Mason Nursing Research Committee of the National Florence Nightingale Memorial Committee of Great Britain and Northern Ireland, London

* In the context of the paper it is relevant to note that all the above single-author research reports were produced by nurses and a nurse was co-author of reference 19.

[18] JOHNSON, J.E. (1972) Effects of structuring patients expectations on their reactions to threatening events. *Nursing Research 21*, 499–504

[19] GILMORE, M. BRUCE, N. & HUNT, M. (1974) *The Work of the Nursing Team in General Practice*, Council for the Education and Training of Health Visitors, London

[20] TIERNEY, A.J. (1975) *Toilet Training Tape/Slide*, University of Edinburgh, Audio Visual Services Department

[21] PRESENT STATE AND FUTURE NEEDS OF GENERAL PRACTICE (1973) *Journal of the Royal College of General Practitioners*, Report No. 16

[22] EDITORIAL (1974) A nurse practitioner. *Lancet 1*, 608–609

[23] DEPARTMENT OF HEALTH AND SOCIAL SECURITY (1974) *Report of the Working Party on Social Work Support for the Health Service*, pp. 22–23, HMSO, London

[24] RUBIN, I.M., PLOVNICK, M.S. & FRY, R.E. (1969) *Improving the Coordination of Care: A Program for Health Team Development*, Ballinger, Cambridge, Massachussetts

Some quandaries facing the health visitor in these times of change

MARY McCLYMONT

Department of Social Science, Stevenage College of Further Education

Abstract Several dilemmas face personnel in the National Health Service as they endeavour to provide quality care while both costs and the level of consumer expectation rise. Amongst the specific aspects of concern to the health visitor are, in particular, role perceptions and role expansion, the problems consequent upon the integration of preventive workers within traditionally curative settings, the perplexities of those concerned with the rightful deployment of skills and resources within the primary health care team, and the need to create group cohesion and efficiency against a background of different professional cultural heritages.

The changing pattern of disease raises several issues, in particular the contribution that health visitors might make to the total health care system.

The overall aim is to examine a few of the areas where there may be conflict and to look at the way in which such conflicts could be harnessed for further cooperation and communication, so improving group harmony and community health care.

Having been associated with the education and training of health visitors and district nurses for over 15 years, during which time the pattern of health care has changed considerably, I find the challenge presented by reorganization of the National Health Service both exciting and a little daunting. It was, therefore, with some trepidation that I began to examine some of the opportunities and incertitude facing the health visitor.

If I were to imply that the health visitor is alone in feeling somewhat perplexed as she views her work within an integrated service, I should give a totally false impression. A recent publication from the Office of Health Economics[1] examines the predicament of *all* health service personnel attempting to meet increasing consumer demand in the face of soaring costs and dwindling resources. The problem of how far social problems can be allowed to continue to become medical problems without some redefinition of medical care is a vexing matter for administrative and professional staffs alike. The conflict of ethics and economics is well demonstrated in daily decision-making, particularly within a hospital.

The question of how to ensure full value in terms of quality of care for money expended could dominate our thinking throughout the symposium but I do not intend to dwell on such aspects. Rather, I shall consider some of the uncertainties that students and colleagues frequently express, many of which have already been well documented, to try to see whether these dilemmas are shared or peculiar to the health visitor. They may be grouped into the following categories:

(1) the effective deployment of skills and resources;
(2) priority ratings and the competing claims of routine and selective visiting —generalism as compared to specialism;
(3) team work in primary health care;
(4) setting goals in primary care.

THE EFFECTIVE DEPLOYMENT OF SKILLS AND RESOURCES

The questions of how best to use limited time and which skills are most profitable to exercise are ones that all health personnel must face. But for many, the problem of the deployment of skills and resources may be easily solved because their work is well delineated and their function is well defined. For the health visitor such decisions are perhaps more difficult, because the limits to her work are much more diffuse. Like her colleague the health education officer, the health visitor sees the whole community as her potential clientele.

Traditionally, the central task of the health visiting service has been regarded as the health care of mothers and young children. Research such as the Greater London Council's study on the work of health visitors in London[2] and June Clark's descriptive analysis of health visiting in Berkshire[3] confirms that most time *is* spent with families with young children, but it would be wrong to assume that the focus of care is entirely upon children, since they may merely provide the *entrée* to a household. Once in contact with a family, health visitors may delve into parental health matters, interpersonal, marital and psychiatric difficulties, housing, social and legal problems and specific needs associated with a state of vulnerability (such as that in single-parent families, handicap, adolescence or middle age). Current statistics show that more of the health visitor's time is now being spent with other groups, particularly the elderly, the chronically sick, the disabled and the bereaved. This substantial minority tends to need more attention and more complex action. Such trends are welcomed by most health visitors but they imply shifts of emphasis from primary to secondary and tertiary levels of prevention.* The present field force of health visitors (equivalent to about 8000 full-time visitors) is hard put to provide quality care to these other age groups without detriment to the families with young children who so obviously need continuing advice and support. One solution to the problem certainly lies in determining what constitutes a realistic case load and working towards its establishment, but although the recommendation by the Department of Health and Social Security[4] of one health visitor for every 3500 in the population is welcomed, it is difficult to discover the evidence on which this figure is based.

Another solution lies in ensuring that only those tasks needing their special skills are undertaken by health visitors. Studies such as those already quoted indicate that health visitors spend about 36% of their time on general administrative work, but many do not have secretarial or clerical help for routine tasks. Accustomed to policy restrictions and to economic stringencies, many workers hesitate to press their legitimate claims for ancillary help. An awareness of the needs of a wide range of vulnerable groups has been created within the profession, and current education and training attempts to provide the specific and unique blend of skills that will enable health visitors to do their defined jobs of health promotion, prevention of disease, the detection and prompt referral of any abnormality amongst the people they visit, health education and supportive care. It is frustrating and perplexing for personnel to find their professional skills underused in the face of pressing medicosocial needs, partly because their time and energy are expended on tasks which, although necessary, could well be done by less highly trained workers. Well might health visitors ask, when will the time be considered ripe for the pyramidal team concept to be developed for health visiting, as Miss Hockey has discussed so clearly?[5]

PRIORITIES AND THE COMPETING CLAIMS OF ROUTINE AND SELECTIVE VISITING

Closely associated with the question of how to safeguard professional time and skills is the decision: where, and how best, to operate?

The original health visitors were envisaged as health missioners and their task defined as visiting the homes of the people to teach the principles of health and the prevention of disease. That Florence Nightingale saw their work as

---

* *Primary prevention*: the process whereby healthy development is encouraged and those influences which contribute to ill-health are identified and minimized; *secondary prevention*: the process whereby established disease is detected early and its duration shortened as far as possible through prompt referral and treatment; *tertiary prevention*: the process whereby after-care is provided with the intention of limiting or containing the effects of a disorder.

encompassing the whole community and being largely home-based is clear from her writings, such as *Sick Nursing and Health Nursing*.[6]

The economic and social events in the UK from 1862 to 1948 led to those early health missioners having their identity linked, first, with the Sanitary Reform Campaign and then, around the turn of the century, with the powerful Maternal and Child Welfare Movement. The deflection of some of their activities into clinics and, from 1907 on, into the schools, although strengthening some of the group educational and advisory aspects of their work, tended to diminish slightly the home health missioner role.

The establishment of the National Health Service in 1948 gave an opportunity for the wider functions of health visiting to be recognized and paved the way for the reappraisal of the role of health visitors in 1953 by the Jameson Committee. When this working party made its report in 1956,[7] it reasserted the claims of health visitors to be regarded as general purpose family visitors with responsibility for preventive medicosocial work. The primary activities were seen to be 'health education and social advice'. The unique feature of health visiting was declared to be its continuity of service within all sections of the community. The relationship between health visitors and families, whether at times of crisis or not, was seen to give an unrivalled opportunity for the study of the normal and for the detection of deviation, so that prompt referral could be made and appropriate action taken. Amongst many points strongly made, the dependence of service efficiency on the ability to survey the whole field at risk stands out. The importance of *regular routine visiting* was emphasized, whether for health teaching, identification of need, or the provision of supportive care. In the changes after some of the recommendations of the report had been accepted, these tenets were constantly re-affirmed.

The setting up in 1962 of a new statutory body (The Council for the Training of Health Visitors) led to a revision of the pattern of preparation of health visitors and of the syllabus of examination. Teaching was broadened, particularly in relation to the behavioural sciences, and efforts were made to educate students for the wider role, whether in traditional administrative settings or newer fields. Steadily rising recruitment is making up the deficit experienced in staffing establishment during the 1950s and if maintained at about 2000 trainees per annum should compensate for the natural loss caused by the retirement of many senior workers.

However, these improvements and the readiness to widen the scope of activity have created further problems for the health visitor. For primary prevention to be effective all sections of the community must be reached regularly, preferably within their own environment; but, except for child care, when the notification of birth leads to prompt visiting, the machinery for contacting other groups is poorly established. Yet, paradoxically, the versatility of the health visitor and the recognition of the contribution she can make at secondary and tertiary preventive levels tend to militate against the home-based primary preventive element of her work. Geographical mobility, with the consequent isolation of small nuclear families and the increasing number of young parents or single elderly people without extended family support, underlines the need for continuing routine surveillance. If this is neglected, health education cannot be offered at the best times; small difficulties which would be easily solved tend to become exaggerated; 'screening' for abnormality tends to be limited, and problems such as child abuse may go undetected in their early stages. Even so, the health visitor is under great pressure to reduce the amount of routine home visiting and operate more selectively. Research has highlighted the needs of more and more vulnerable groups, such as families with handicapped children,[8-11] single-parent families,[12] those experiencing emotional or social deprivation,[13, 14] those suffering prolonged or terminal illness[15] or bereavement.[16] Health visitors are aware that, with their medical, nursing and social work colleagues, they can contribute to the care of such families but, unless the profession can be expanded rapidly, concentration on selective visiting may leave the routine work undone with undesirable consequences.

The need to increase recruitment for health visitors even more presents further problems, since the nature and breadth of the work demand several entry qualifications and comprehensive preparation of the recruit. These requirements in their turn mean that there must be enough suitable entrants to nursing and that the standard of nurses' education must be high at various stages of basic and post-registration preparation. The present revised basic training for nurses is helping towards an awareness of the importance of nursing in community health, but the delay and confusion over reform of nursing education are having serious repercussions.

GENERALIST AND SPECIALIST DUTIES

How far health visitors should continue to cling to their generalist function presents a further dilemma. The need for some specialization is strongly advocated by those who recognize the claims by specific groups for expert knowledge and care but it is feared that, if the traditional general nature of the work is reduced, the continuity of family health care may be lost. Reforms within the social services have led to a generic approach in social work instead of specialization and this has confused the issue still further.[15]

Possibly, the answer lies in the formation of a larger body of generalist health visitors within general medical practice, with a cadre of specialist health visitors who are able to offer their expertise over a wider geographical location.

DILEMMAS OF TEAM WORK FOR PRIMARY HEALTH CARE

Administrative changes have set further problems for the health visitor. Since the 1950s general practitioners, district nurses and health visitors have been generally working closer together, mostly to great advantage. The early schemes demonstrated the benefits of such partnership: the wider scope of work and the improvements in standard of care resulting from the doctor, nurse or health visitor being more fully informed of a patient's medical or psychosocial state. Then, there was generally a commitment to collaborate and communicate. The success of these pioneer ventures led to their wider adoption; current statistics show that about 78% of health visitors and 72% of district nurses work within general medical practice. However, the mere adoption of an administrative measure does not constitute acceptance of the philosophy of team work. For several groups, it is clear they have merely transferred their traditional skills into a new framework. Without the commitment to collaboration, which characterized the pilot schemes, the primary health care team remains in many instances only a collection of individuals.

The monograph published by the Council for the Education and Training of Health Visitors[17] on the work of the nursing team in general practice shows that, although nurses in the 39 teams studied were unanimous about the advantages of team work with general practitioners, several factors cause serious disquiet. Although, theoretically, opportunities for closer cooperation and communication exist, in practice in most teams 'there was a *laissez-faire* approach adopted by members in regard to contact with each other ... most teams seemed to be composed of small cells of colleagues from the same discipline ... More of the General Practitioners and District Nurses were satisfied with the *laissez-faire* approach to communication, than were the health visitors who regard their work as lacking in integration with their colleagues ...' The dilemma of the health visitor is thus posed: poised on the edge of health, social and educational work and often aware of the importance of both a free flow of communication and group dynamics, she is faced with the need to encourage regular purposeful meetings with colleagues who may be reluctant to give more time to such activities. If she accepts chance consultations and *ad hoc* discussion arrangements, then she may lose the opportunity to promote useful regular contact. If she presses the issue she may further jeopardize a tenuous relationship.

To many doctors the role of the health visitor is shadowy and imprecise. They are not accustomed to working with a nursing practitioner who initiates the bulk of her own work. This is easy to understand. Medical training focuses largely on curing. The relationship between doctor and nurse is perceived largely in terms of the hospital functions, with marked differences of status and clearly defined tasks. Both doctor and nurse can appreciate the complementary nature of their work, and their interdependence. Even though they may not always have had close administrative links in the past, general practitioners have always been aware of the contribution of district nurses. They have referred patients for care and nurses in turn have expected medical treatment to be prescribed.

Traditionally, the health visitor has worked with a community rather than focusing on the needs of one client. Her role is more one of finding cases than of accepting cases. Far from relieving the general practitioner's work-load, she is likely to increase it and, if she works successfully, she will be seeking to increase his preventive orientation. The misunderstandings which can so easily arise thus need more time and opportunity for discussion. But if the health visitor wants to encourage harmonious working relationships she may fear to arouse controversy and so may avoid airing difficulties. Current health visiting education stresses the 'enabling function' of the health visitor within the team; she facilitates colleagues in their professional tasks but, when district nurses and general practitioners do not always understand some of the non-technical aspects of the work of health visitors, they may be less able to reciprocate. General practitioners and district nurses not only have clearly perceived roles, they also have recognized tools for their tasks. The health visitor, with her more ambiguous duties, needs different but equally important tools. These include age–sex registers, vulnerability indexes and access to family health profiles, hospital referral records etc. As the machinery for forging these tools lies mainly outside the control of the health visitor, she often depends on the goodwill and service of the secretarial staff within a general practice. If she presses her claims too vigorously she may be viewed as demanding and disruptive; if she fails to press them, she cannot function effectively! The dilemma is obvious.

WORK IN CLINICS

An increasingly important feature of modern general practice is the development of a wider range of activities in clinics. These offer great opportunities for collaborative work between team members and hold great promise for the future. But health visitors, who traditionally operated over a large geographical area, have become identified with a community clinic and, although more doctors are tending to hold antenatal, postnatal or child health clinics at their practice premises, several clients still use the community clinic which may be situated nearer to them. Health visitors running such clinics are likely to meet clients registered with several different practices and, unless they try to collaborate frequently with other doctors and health visitors, there is a risk that the information available will not be adequate, with the result that conflicting advice may be given. This dilemma has been highlighted recently by Brimblecombe *et al.* in their report *Bridging in Health*.[18] If the health visitor concentrates wholly on building up clinics in the practice she may lose contact with clients and staff in community clinics and the school health service. Furthermore, the organization of social work teams, which are based in the community and work within a defined geographical area, may mean that the health visitor is at a disadvantage when dealing with community affairs. Any attempt to retain this close community contact, which is so valuable, demands extra time and effort. If the health visitor decides not to foster the development of practice-based clinics she may lose valuable opportunities for mutual help and cooperation in patient care.

GOAL-SETTING IN PRIMARY HEALTH CARE

The concept of primary health care is currently receiving world-wide attention, not only because of its economic implications, but also because of psychological and sociological factors. So far there is limited evidence of systematic identification by teams of the aims and objectives in primary health care. This makes evaluation difficult.

The desirability of egalitarian working relationships is now being actively promoted by nursing managers and educators. Yet differences in status and traditional attitudes create more difficulties for the nurses in the team than for the medical and social workers. Health visitors less accustomed to the 'handmaiden role' than their nursing colleagues in hospitals are likely to want to be more vocal in their demands for group decisions about what is to be prevented, controlled, treated or restored and/or who is to be supported. Consequently, they may initially undermine the cohesion of the group by pointing out areas of conflict. Members of the team must get together and work out common policies for programmes of preventive and supportive care. Attention will have to turn from treatment of episodic illness to dealing with the chronic disabling conditions and behavioural disorders. These changes in the pattern of working will demand new skills and different attitudes. Both interdisciplinary and multidisciplinary training during service will be necessary and the strengths and weaknesses of the group will have to be analysed. The tasks of retaining professional identity, developing role awareness in respect of self and others and ensuring maximum flexibility and cooperation will not be easy.

The British Medical Association's report[19] sets our certain components for the success of primary health care teams but emphasizes that making the necessary bids for resources, collecting appropriate data and devising effective schemes will demand tactical skills and working strategies.

Health visitors as well as other nursing team members ought to remember the famous dictum of their predecessor Florence Nightingale: 'Reports are not self-executive'. Should they wait for general practitioners to take the initiative?

Over the past 20 years, health visitors have demonstrated a tremendous capacity for coping with change. They have adopted a totally new approach to their education and training, broadening the syllabus and altering the pattern of examination, under the general guidance of a new statutory body. They have introduced field-work teachers, accepted male entrants into their profession, and have initiated research into practice.

Because of their regular contact with all sections of the community they are ideally placed to detect the hopes and fears and observe the health needs of the public. They not only have the chance to involve the community in health matters, working closely with self-help groups, but are in a particularly advantageous position to identify and interpret the needs of the many inarticulate individuals who may well be experiencing great stress in the present unstable society. In exploring some of their dilemmas it is important not to lose sight of the positive contribution that the profession is making and can continue to make. How far the current quandaries can be used for progress will depend on certain factors. The profession must make up its own mind about the perimeter of its field of work. The respective roles of social workers and health visitors may need to be clarified, perhaps as a result of action research. Nursing management can help to remedy some of the working conditions. But the understanding and positive help of medical and nursing colleagues could go a long way towards dispelling some of the present difficulties, so that by further modification of their attitudes and regular evaluation of their work health visitors may find their own answers to some of their current perplexities.

Discussion

Gollan: In the general practice unit which I organize we have almost 100% attachment of community services—health visitors, geriatric visitors, social workers and district nurse. The group started about 25 years ago with a nurse attached, and the partners always aimed to have a health visitor. When in 1965 the London County Council broke up, we finally secured the attachment of a health visitor and then a district nurse—we now have even an age–sex register! Soon after the health visitor and social worker were attached, they altered the pattern of work and organization in the practice, but we did not consider them to be 'militant' on this account. They quickly objected to conducting all their negotiations with the general practitioners on the stairs, in corridors and so on; this they felt was most unsatisfactory, and so did the general practitioners. We therefore instituted something which has now become a focal part of our practice organization, namely a weekly meeting of every member of the team, including receptionists, secretaries and district nurse, to discuss not only health visiting or social work problems, but other matters, such as practice policy. This has been enormously valuable. At no time did we feel that the health visitor was interrupting our work but rather that she was developing it.

With regard to interdisciplinary teaching, we have a continuous attachment of all sorts of students (medical students, nursing students, health visitor students, social work students) to our centre and the general practitioners in our unit aim to hold interdisciplinary seminars. In practice this does not always succeed because the students' programmes sometimes do not fit in but, where we have managed it, the experience has been valuable. Medical students particularly get a tremendous feedback from at least some teaching with members of other groups.

If anybody should think that as a result of the attachment of these additional workers the doctors have less to do, they are wrong—all our partners maintain that Parkinson's Law operates: the more people there are delving into the problems of patients and trying to improve the care, the more is uncovered and, if anything, we are involved in more work.

Tait: General practice needs health visitors desperately. At the same time as educating patients, the health visitor will educate general practitioners and *vice versa.*

Roberts: Since the reorganization of the health service, a vacuum has existed where prevention used to be. The Public Health Service has gone and the School Health Service is in disarray. Community medicine is responsible for the organization and delivery of *all* medical services and its involvement with prevention, *per se,* is both small and tangential. Those who organized this new service seem to have assumed that new generations of clinicians will become just as enthusiastic about prevention as they currently are about cure. This assumption remains to be proven. Practice of the preventive philosophy needs the application of skills, motivations and temperament to professional objectives which are, in many ways, distinct from those required in clinical practice. If my contention that it may be too difficult in future to incorporate into one doctor the dual motivation of clinical and preventive practice contains some truth, the future service may become largely clinically oriented and the impetus for prevention lost.

Hockey: One of the main problems in primary care is that possibly no member of the team finds it easy to evaluate their efficiency or effectiveness. On what basis does one judge a team to be a good team? Prevention cannot be measured easily. Health visitors are hard put to evaluate their own performance; some assess it in terms of the number of visits, the number of children immunized or the number of other achievements. This is not always helpful. Having been a health visitor tutor myself, I know that health visitors sometimes can make a genuine and sincere effort to demonstrate what can be done by a health visitor; but they may, in doing so, create problem families—that may sound facetious but it is only too easy. All families have problems and the distinction between a family with a problem and a problem family often lies in the eye of the beholder, the health visitor.

Roy: Isn't it true that the functions of the health visitor are nebulously defined? They overlap with those of the district nurse (many of whose tasks are appropriate to an enrolled nurse) and they blur into those of the social workers who, at present, are having great problems mainly due to inadequate experience and training. We ought to think again about community nursing[20] and take the opportunity of the Briggs report[21] to consider how the various aspects of community nursing should be covered in the future by altering the patterns of training to suit particular tasks in the various areas as well as by defining the limits of the tasks of each group.

Bickerton: I cannot accept that the district nurse does the work of enrolled nurses. When surgical patients are discharged, whom do you want to care for them?

Roy: An enrolled nurse would change dressings, remove sutures, etc., very well.

Bickerton: There must be a state registered nurse, the equivalent of a nursing sister, in the district. I agree that enrolled nurses could undertake minor nursing procedures. If we are going to maintain high standards of nursing and consider early discharge from hospitals, with consequently more care in the community (a particularly relevant point now [i.e. December 1975], when patients are not being admitted to hospital unless they are considered to be emergencies and so the bulk of the work is being invested firmly in the community), we must have qualified nurses responsible for the nursing care. We have auxiliaries and enrolled nurses to help.

The role of the community nurse covers prevention and cure for all age groups. What are her priorities? She will put curative work before prevention if she has a heavy case load—that is only human nature. This is what happens with midwifery and general care; health visiting comes second or third best.

The health visitor is in a dilemma: before she is seconded to a group, she knows one area extremely well but, as general practitioners have patients spread all across a town or district, she now spends much more time behind the steering wheel of a car. Previously, her knowledge of the area enabled her to notice details such as a change of curtains or the appearance of nappies on washing lines but now the family she knows might be registered with another practice. Why cannot general practitioners consider zoning themselves—even if only for the sake of the petrol consumption?

Roy: I was not suggesting abolition of the district nurse but rather that we should look at her functions—at present the enrolled nurse could perform many of them. The community nurse is not the health visitor with another name; she could have a clinical role as well as one of education and prevention. The restructuring of training that the Briggs report suggested would make appropriate training easier and provide an opportunity that will facilitate change, although the report itself still sees a distinction between 'family clinical (home nursing) and family health (health visiting) services'.[21]

Hockey: A district nurse does not perform tasks, she looks after patients. An enrolled nurse may be able to do a dressing for one person, but giving an injection to someone who is vulnerable to depression, say, should be the job of the registered nurse because she would recognize the vulnerability. We should emphasize patient-oriented care, not task-oriented care.

Tait: We have been asked to define our goals in terms of what can be beaten and what has to be borne, which is a useful distinction. General practitioners see the pressures in 20th century medicine as being more about chronic disease and old age. This is where we see the needs of our society pressing on the medical services. We understand why health visitors have concentrated on the care of children but we must now ask whether so much skill and energy should be channelled in that direction. Health visitors, too, have to analyse their goals, and perhaps redefine some of them.

Birley: I am reminded of the apocryphal comment of the child watching the film *Quo Vadis*: 'One poor lion hasn't got a Christian'. I am puzzled why health visitors are feeling so deprived, because with a population of about 50 million, 8000 full-time health visitors should each have a case-load of about 450 children under five years of age. If they now want to take on old people as well, they must be seriously concerned for themselves. One possible cause of this dissatisfaction could be their 'no-win' position: if a client remains unnoticeably healthy, the health visitor has been doing her job, but if the client becomes noticeably ill, she is seen to have failed.

Knox: Health visitors and also community midwives will find active allies in the new community health councils. In our council we are conscious of the profound and comprehensive knowledge of the community which health visitors and midwives have and which neither the council's staff nor its members can approach. Although the National Health Service continues to be dominated by attitudes which are hospital oriented, the establishment of district health care planning teams should ensure a better understanding of community needs, and as an early priority these groups must seek to involve people working in primary care and prevention.

Guz: I am amazed that health visitors are wondering about their role. As our concern for prevention covers clinical and sub-clinical disease, the detection of, for instance, asymptomatic hypertension would mean taking the blood pressure of everybody in the community. That one example implies the need for a vast number of workers, far greater than the present corps.

McClymont: It is not that health visitors are worried about whether their role will continue but rather that, because the skills they can offer can be used by many vulnerable groups, they face the difficulty of knowing where to set the boundaries when not all the demands can be met. Prevention has suddenly become a fashionable concept but, as Dr Roberts pointed out, the administrative machinery for a fully preventive service has been removed. Health visitors have to fight hard to safeguard their primary preventive role. The enormity of the task and the increased diversification of function has forced health visitors to become more concerned about how effective they are.

Elliott: Ought not the vastness of the task of prevention be thought about in terms of its component parts and possible delegation? The nursing auxiliary has already been mentioned. If we need to measure the blood pressure of everybody in the community, surely people could be quickly trained just to take blood pressures in the way that thousands of lay people in China were trained to do the necessary blood tests, etc., when the decision was made to stamp out venereal disease?[22]

McClymont: A pyramidal team is needed but, as we have heard, we are not sure which way the pyramid works. Devolution of tasks is vital; 36% of the health visitor's time is now spent on routine administrative work which could easily be delegated but the resources have not been made available to us. The health visitor's skills are the most underutilized in the whole nursing profession. This is one of the problems we face.

Russell: And it will remain as long as the priorities of the health visitor are decided by somebody who has no preventive orientation. Most health boards are not asking what problems should and can be prevented in the long term but rather what types of prevention are effective. Thus, a shift from primary to secondary and tertiary prevention is likely because the effects of the last two are immediate and easier to see.

Huntingford: We have heard that nurses need patients. Now we hear that health visitors are looking for jobs. I must return to my earlier question: 'do people need us?' We shall not solve the problem if we start to look for tasks to do. We must determine how much can be done effectively with existing skills and then decide where we can best exercise them. We pay lip service to consumer participation. Instead of defining our jobs in terms of consumer needs, we define them in terms of our satisfaction and what we can do to make our lives better. I am fed up with this selfish preoccupation, which is symptomatic of our present problems. Doctors are currently [i.e. December 1975] making people do without them, and are almost admitting that they can do without people. I am very glad that nurses need people, but do people need us?

Arie: I, too, am puzzled by this vacuum which we are trying to fill. In my work, chiefly in the psychiatry of the elderly, there is a mammoth task for health visitors in which we find them eagerly participating. At Goodmayes Hospital we have come to rely more on nurses who work with the patients at home and to develop supportive networks. At present, we have no less than five such networks of nurses: health visitors; district nurses; 'community psychiatric nurses' based outside the hospital; 'community nurses' based in the hospital and working outwards from the hospital; and ward nurses, who are increasingly keen to extend their work outside the hospital, by following up their patients or even by seeing them before admission. Within these networks, I am sometimes uneasy about who should be doing what, which nurses should be helping whom. We probably now need some rationalization of these competing and complementary networks (there is no shortage of work for them all). Or perhaps it is just intolerance of pluralism on my part! The eagerness to get people out of hospitals is certainly matched by the eagerness of nurses to look after them outside hospital.

Bridger: With the growing need to deal effectively with increasing interdependence, whether interdisciplinary or community-based, we shall have to learn how to operate in network systems. For instance, *everyone* relevant to a particular situation is involved in the managing of overlapping and conflicting interests and not just the executive figure, as in the more simple hierarchical structures.

McClymont: A strength of the health visiting service is the continuity of its care. However, once a large range of activities and opportunities for service is presented, many workers enter that field. There is a danger that this may negate continuity of care. When, for example, because of pressure of work from other groups, the health visitor is diverted from working with under-fives and their parents, there is a proliferation of other workers such as the 'parent educator' or the pre-school play adviser, who may visit homes. If the health visitor does not work with the over 65s then a 'geriatric visitor' is introduced—similarly with the mentally disordered and visiting psychiatric community nurses. The moment that the health visitor or another professional worker becomes aware of how she can contribute to the care of other vulnerable groups she is faced with this problem of maintaining a continuing caring service which is not just related to crisis. The urgent need is for an increase in the health visiting work force; this would solve our problems.

Bickerton: The health visitor is not short of work; we carry tremendous case-loads of work almost from family planning or conception to bereavement. As Miss McClymont mentioned, the Jameson report[7] recommended one health visitor to every 4300 people (and more recently this has been reduced to 3500 people), but at present it is more like one to 6000–7000 people and often more within general practice. Our loyalties are torn; we are basically nurses who have been drawn into social work by general practitioners since the reorganization, but we are not recognized as social workers. We are now more of a buffer between the two, in addition to our role as educators.

Baderman: The patient is by no means the least confused in all this. Some do not know who visited them and can hardly remember whether they said the same thing to each of them. Then the doctors have to find out who is going to turn off the gas, feed the canary or whatever on their behalf.

Roy: Are we not restating the question of what do the people want? If we consider people, we must consider families, and it seems a basic principle that a family should have two people only to whom they refer for advice about any aspect of their health: a doctor and a nurse. In terms of those available for community care, would it not be generally more advantageous to have each person looking after a few families but covering a wide range of their needs than to have many people looking after the specific needs of many families?

Bridger: We are beginning to face some of the options that are open to us for some of the problems that have been defined. We seem to be thinking in terms of Schumacher's 'small-is-beautiful' rather than the large institution designed on an 'economy-of-scale' basis.

Birley: In addition to his skills, we should consider what a professional worker is empowered to do. Social workers, like doctors, can initiate the compulsory removal of children and adults from their homes to 'places of care'. They don't use this power often. I wonder whether health visitors or others would want such power to cope with vulnerable families.

Baderman: Dr Roy's suggestion is inherently attractive but it seems that the tendency towards increased specialization in all groups is working against it. People opt to be health visitors, community-based nurses, geriatric nurses and so on; it may prove difficult to put the clock back, however desirable that may be.

Roy: The community nurse could be protected from being monopolized by curative work by restricting the number of families under her care. She would then have time for education and prevention with these families. Having more time, she would have the *entrée* in the curative area and then expand into prevention and *vice versa*.

Beckhard: A multiplicity of loyalties is the price one has to pay for working in a multi-task profession. This discussion indicates that the choice of professionals, such as home visitors, nurses and others, to do several tasks is being removed. The issue may become how to manage the complexity rather than how to make it disappear.

Roy: From a practical point of view, the training programme for community nurses at enrolled level in Kenya (particularly at Kisumu) proved to be a great success. Although it operates in a different economic environment to that in this country, it is relevant. These girls, basically generalist community nurses, are most useful and complete the nucleus of the primary care team of medical assistant, health inspector and nurse with the district physician and registered (graduate) nurse in support.

Hockey: Both Miss McClymont and I have worked in a village setting; it can be most satisfying, if the case-load is small enough. Also, health teaching is more effective if patients have or have had a pathological condition which makes the teaching relevant to them.

Bridger: Whereas one might point to the village as being the past, it may yet be the stage to which we must return, although perhaps in a different way. Dr Roy's comments can then be taken as looking forward towards network systems in which one can have both a generalist function and a more direct specialist affiliation, while being part of a small-but-beautiful entity in a larger whole.

Beckhard: In the USA the wave of specialism has reached its peak and the age of technology as an end in itself seems to be passing. Both legislation and public values are moving towards more generalism with greater emphasis on primary, ambulatory care, education and service. Probably within a couple of years medical schools will have to train 50% of their students as general practitioners, if they are to get government or financial support for them.

Joyson: I advocate a resocialization programme for the country before we go ahead with the provision of more services. First, society is such that we are led to believe that family units have broken up for a variety of reasons and are no longer self-supportive and, further, that the major problem in psychiatric, geriatric and, increasingly, general hospitals is social—the placement of patients fit for discharge who have nowhere to go. By resocialization I mean that families should be more willing to accept responsibility, wherever possible, for their relatives who need to be looked after; if they were, we would have fewer of these problems.

Arie: I must challenge that. Families are on the whole impressively supportive. Some 95% of old people are at home. Successive surveys of the burden that is left on families by the statutory services reveal the colossal burden that families had been carrying even *before* they approached the services.[23] We tend to be egocentric about this, asking, are we doing enough for families? But it is amazing what families do *not* ask for help with. Most families may take it less for granted that they should give total care but, in the context of present-day expectations of the good life, it is astonishing that they still do so much for their dependent relatives; they are certainly not rejecting them.

Another polarity that is becoming apparent is between generalism and specialism. Both specialists and generalists have tasks which they do better than the other. It is not an either/or choice. Let us bear in mind, too, that the cosy image of the generalist giving comprehensive care—the general practitioner, the nurse, the social worker—can be oppressive by binding the client or family into a single relationship from which they cannot escape. It is a commonplace for people working in hospitals that patients will frequently seek one out because they want to make certain transactions with one and not with their general practitioner, precisely because he knows them so well. They may at times want to escape from this binding, even paternalistic, system of total family support. Total care does have tremendous virtues, but people must have an opportunity to deal with others, to have an element of choice or escape, such as may be provided through seeing the specialist.

Roberts: Certain views that have been expressed so far seem to support my point that practitioners of clinical and of preventive medicine tend to operate from different premises. The health visitor wants to see people who are *well* and to prevent them from becoming ill; in contrast, Dr Guz refers to prevention in *patients*. The clinician is always likely to be drawn towards detecting illness in order to treat the patient because only in these circumstances can he use his substantial diagnostic skills. Prevention of ill health in people who are well demands neither complex diagnostic facilities nor complicated therapeutic procedures. Thus in the practice of true prevention, the doctor is unable to exercise those skills which he has acquired after a long and arduous training.

Tait: Is this division between preventive and clinical medicine as real as we imagine? Consider the historical development of health visiting. The task of health visitors was first defined in relation to a clinical situation very different from today's. Amongst children, the incidence of preventable diseases like rickets was high and the children were denied access to adequate primary medical care. The pay-off for work with this group was then high. Now the pay-off is much less or, at least, less obvious. Maybe we would do better to find out where clinical medicine is inadequate in other areas and concentrate the work of the health visitor there.

McClymont: If we were to do that we might miss other things, such as battering in children.

Guz: My sympathies and experience lie entirely with what Mr Joyson said. Anglo-Saxon and Scandinavian culture contains a considerable amount of family rejection. In many hospitals about 20–30% of the beds may be occupied by patients fit for discharge but with nowhere to go. Dr Arie cannot say that families are performing their function well in our culture. In India, families —admittedly, sometimes large families—show a completely different attitude to the sick and to caring. In Mediterranean and Muslim cultures, too, the attitude is different. After 25 years of medical practice I am sure that the relationship between the elderly sick and their relatives is deteriorating, although that is hard to prove.

Russell: Positive rejection differs from the lack of the capacity to care. The changes in social structure have led to a decrease in the capacity to care; families are smaller and more mobile than before, more wives are working. For such reasons, many cannot give as much care now.

Roy: When one looks at urban communities in East Africa, such as in Nairobi, old people who could not be looked after were beginning to become a problem. The relatives were worried, but they had moved into a small house (usually shared) or a flat in the city, and the flat or house was already overcrowded. In the country districts there would have been no problem: the old person could have lived in another hut. It is no different in this country really. The problems are largely with old people who physically cannot be looked after or who would totally disrupt a family if brought back into it. I am more optimistic and believe that we are assisting families who need assistance and that few evade their responsibilities.

Arie: We are now at the centre of UK health needs in a changing setting. Dr Guz described some of the attitudes which are so inappropriate to the present-day pattern of need for health services; the rejection of old people is not so much by families as by health professionals. The placement problem ('disposal') is only what one sees as a disposal problem. The figures are eloquent: at any one time, in round figures, 95% of people over 65 are at home, 1% are in general and geriatric hospitals, 1% are in mental hospitals, 2% are in old people's homes and 1% are in various other places. The 2% in hospitals account for nearly half the beds in the National Health Service. Whether one regards these people as disposal problems who should be looked after by their families, or by someone else, or as legitimate users of the resources of one's own sector of the health service is also a question of attitudes. Our attitudes in a changing setting have to adapt to the realities—namely, that the health service now exists largely to care for the elderly and the chronically ill. Our job as professionals is in almost every specialty more and more concerned with such problems, and with underpinning the care which families are giving.

Baderman: A less emotive example than that of 'disposal' of the elderly is the marked change in attitude among both the 'clients' in the population and the dispensers of health care towards using large and complex medical organizations for the provision of medical care. One can exemplify that with accidents and emergencies. The client considers that it is no longer right, desirable, safe or morally acceptable either to treat an abrasion at home or to take it to a general practitioner or, if he does, a substantial number of reputable and responsible general practitioners believe that it is a matter for the hospital, not general practice. Cultural changes, or changes in habits, are altering the way in which medical care is 'doled out' in the acute sphere as well as in the geriatric sphere. This is common at least throughout North-West Europe, where 'minor' and 'major' acute medical problems are being shifted not only from the community-based emergency care services into hospital-based services but into increasingly larger hospital-based services. Nobody has yet proved whether it is better, more efficient or more economic to do so. This trend can be seen at its most extreme in Paris where not only do practitioners and small hospitals not provide emergency care and the public do not want them to, but the hospitals must now have helicopter parks, because even ambulances are not really 'the thing' nowadays. If we are not careful it may catch on here.

Gollan: About 25 or 30 years ago, was not 'family care' often a euphemism for care by an unmarried daughter in the family? In general practice we encounter middle-aged women who have become psychiatric patients simply because their parents, to whom they have devoted their whole lives at home, have suddenly died and they have no further apparent object in life since they are without profession or job. This has been changed and changed for the better.

Guz: Although Dr Arie and I disagree, neither of us can prove whether families care because we cannot measure care and consequently we cannot determine whether families care. Returning to the problems of the old, I am only saying that unless one considers that there are too many acute medical beds—a view for which there is little evidence—then it seems ridiculous for people to stay in hospital for social reasons at £80–100 a week without any medical reasons. Whether their families can take them back or not, there is a deficit of care in the community. If that is what Dr Arie is saying, I would agree. 20–30% of acute medical beds occupied by those elderly patients are desperately needed for the acute sick—old and young. 'Disposal' is a dreadful, disgraceful word (even if we use it sometimes in desperation.) The point is underlined by visitors from the cultures that I mentioned; when we go to the East we are dismayed by leprosy, when they come here they are dismayed by the way families care for the old.

Nurses sometimes monitor how many visitors patients receive. Even though people work during the day, visiting presumably is the best expression of care; we have a depressingly large number of older patients (not only over 65) in acute medical beds in London hospitals who are rarely or never visited by their young relatives.

Paine: The official solution to the problem of long-stay patients blocking acute medical beds is the community hospital, into which these patients could be admitted if general practitioners like Dr Tait are prepared to look after them there. After all this is how geriatric and long-term care as a separate specialty started—through pressure from general physicians in acute hospitals to unblock their beds.

Baderman: Do you see the community hospital as a move back into the community?

Paine: Some see the community hospital as a second-rate institution but others see it as a way of solving a real problem in a logical fashion.

Huntingford: Although I agree with Dr Guz about cultural differences and the value of extended families, we should not extrapolate from the developing world to judge the quality of our care of the aged. Care of the elderly and infirm is not yet a sizeable problem in developing countries, in which, as Dr Guz pointed out, the size of families is so much greater. It is also misleading to use the number of visitors to the sick as an index of the quality of care. We should not be reported as making a plea on the basis of invalid comparisons for a return to the extended family as a solution to caring for the elderly and chronic sick.

Roy: The chances of ordinary people occupying acute beds during their lifetime are small; if they do, their stay will be about 2–3 weeks. It does not matter whether they stay in a hospital in their town or 50 miles away. If they are going to be in hospital for a prolonged period, they will be suffering from a chronic illness, usually associated with old age, and, if so, they should be nursed in the community, in a community hospital.

References

1 OFFICE OF HEALTH ECONOMICS (1975) *The Health Care Dilemma*, Report No. 53, Office of Health Economics, London
2 MARRIS, T. (1970) *The Work of Health Visitors in London*, Planning and Transportation Research Report No. 12, Greater London Council
3 CLARK, J. (1973) *A Family Visitor*, The Royal College of Nursing, London
4 DEPARTMENT OF HEALTH AND SOCIAL SECURITY (1972) *Aids to Improved Efficiency in the Local Authority Service Deployment of the Nursing Team*, Circular 13/72, HMSO, London
5 HOCKEY, L. (1972) *Use or Abuse: a study of the state enrolled nurse in the local authority nursing services*, Queen's Institute of District Nursing, London
6 NIGHTINGALE, F. (1893) Sick nursing and health nursing, in *Selected Writings of Florence Nightingale* (1954) (compiled by Lucy Ridgeley Seymer), MacMillan, New York
7 MINISTRY OF HEALTH, DEPARTMENT OF HEALTH FOR SCOTLAND AND MINISTRY OF EDUCATION (1956) *An Inquiry into Health Visiting*, Working Party on The Field of Work, Training and Recruitment of Health Visitors (Chairman Sir W. Jameson), HMSO, London
8 YOUNGHUSBAND, E. *et al.* (1970) *Living with Handicap* (Davie, R., Birchall, D. & Pringle, M.L.K., eds.) National Bureau for Co-operation in Child Care, London
9 MCMICHAEL, J.K. (1971) *Handicap: a study of physically handicapped children and their families*, Staples Press, London
10 HEWETT, S. (1970) *The Family and The Handicapped Child*, Allen and Unwin, London
11 FOX, M. (1974) *They Get This Training But They Don't Know How You Feel*, The Association for Action for the Crippled Child, London
12 HUNT, A., FOX, J. & MORGAN, M. (1973) *Families and Their Needs*, vol. 1 and 2, Office of Population, Censuses and Surveys, Social Survey Division, HMSO, London
13 RUTTER, M. (1966) *The Children of Sick Parents*, Oxford University Press, London
14 PROSSER, H. & WEDGE, P. (1973) *Born to Fail*, Arrow Books, London
15 CARTWRIGHT, A., ANDERSON, J.L. & HOCKEY, L. (1973) *Life Before Death*, Routledge, London
16 PARKES, C.M. & BROWN, R.J. (1972) Health and bereavement. A controlled study of young Boston widows and widowers. *Psychosomatic Medicine 34*, 444–461
17 GILMORE, M., BRUCE, N. & HUNT, M. (1974) *The Work of the Nursing Team in General Practice*, The Council for the Education and Training of Health Visitors, London
18 BRIMBLECOMBE, F.S.W., CARTWRIGHT, K. *et al.* (1975) *Bridging in Health*, Oxford University Press for the Nuffield Hospitals Trust, London
19 BRITISH MEDICAL ASSOCIATION (1974) *Primary Health Care Teams* (Board of Science and Education Report) British Medical Association, London
20 REPORT ON PRIMARY HEALTH CARE TEAMS, BRITISH MEDICAL ASSOCIATION BOARD OF SCIENCE AND EDUCATION (1974) pp. 13–16, British Medical Association, London
21 REPORT OF THE COMMITTEE ON NURSING (BRIGGS REPORT) (1972) Cmnd. 5115, HMSO, London
22 HORN, J.S. (1969) *Away with All Pests: an English surgeon in People's China*, ch. 9, Scribner, New York
23 HAWKS, D. (1975) Community care: an analysis of assumption. *British Journal of Psychiatry, 127*, 276–285

Commitment and concern in the health service

R. D. WEIR

Department of Community Medicine, University of Aberdeen

Abstract   As part of a general review of the use of local health services resources, a specific enquiry was mounted to examine the recurring complaint of a lack of identity or sense of belonging made by staff working in the largest district of the Grampian Health Board.

The investigation pointed to clearly identifiable sources of confusion and concern:

(a) a need to identify with and feel committed to the health service;
(b) a sense of purpose and direction;
(c) satisfaction with the conditions of service;
(d) an understanding of an individual's role and its relationship to others'.

It is relatively easy to list the problems, such as friction between occupational groups, lack of commitment, uncertainty over duties and authority, reluctance to delegate and resistance to, or even outright rejection of, decisions apparently at variance with professional advice.

In addition to these internal stresses the health service is perpetually beset by two other external problems, namely what it is expected to achieve and the finance allowed to attain its goals. The various groups within the service are in no way agreed on roles and responsibilities. Without agreement, goals cannot be defined. Without goals, use of resources cannot be rationalized. Without a demonstrably fair distribution of resources, neither the public nor health service staff will feel confident or committed. Somewhere this cycle must be broken.

A recurring complaint these days is the lack of identity or sense of belonging which is increasingly being expressed by those working in the health service. The issue has been represented as a general malaise affecting all categories of staff but particularly those exposed to the impersonal administration assumed to be associated with large functional units. In addition to obtaining a general view through repeated contacts with staff of several health boards, we had an opportunity to assess the extent and origin of such feelings in a health board district; because of the general nature of the issues explored it is likely that the findings may have a wide application. The district contains 20 hospitals with some 1200 beds in a central complex and employs over 7000 staff. In endeavouring to explore these questions we considered two approaches: (i) an attitude survey covering all categories of staff and (ii) an interview of representatives of as wide a range of staff as possible. Eventually, a modification of the second approach was adopted. The resulting discussions point to clearly identifiable sources of confusion and concern and can most conveniently be considered under the following four headings:

(a) a need to identify with and feel committed to the health service;
(b) a sense of purpose and direction;
(c) satisfaction with the conditions of service;
(d) an understanding of an individual's role and its relationship to others'.

FACTORS CONSIDERED

a) *Commitment to the Health Service*

Perhaps the most encouraging feature of all the conversations was the widespread basic belief in the health service. A commitment certainly exists, but it would be both wrong and unwise to trade on it. The previous unity of the health service is under considerable strain; cultural, social and technical changes have considerably modified the relationships between the various categories of staff and their expectations. As a result, the commitment of both individuals and groups is being eroded and, as in any large organization with a proliferation of consultative and negotiating agencies, militancy (aggression or frustration, whatever word one cares to use) is appearing as a means of both promoting and preventing changes. It is difficult to be objective within a stressed organization and the sense of commitment will only operate effectively when some of the other issues, about to be discussed, have been resolved.

(b) *Purpose and direction within the Service*

Inevitably, during the discussions the question of leadership arose and in the general sense in which it is being used here it is akin to the subject matter of the previous section (a). Not surprisingly, reorganization of the health service has lost its impetus: for three or four years people were working towards or waiting for the event and now that it is past there is an inevitable sense of anticlimax. Previously, integration was to some an impending event as a result of which things would be better and the service would improve, but it appears that despite all the preparation, promotion and publication most staff do not completely understand what has happened or how the new service is intended to operate. Other staff have never appreciated any need for reorganization and have viewed the preparations with foreboding and gloom. For them, not surprisingly, the event has confirmed their prediction of not an anticlimax but a near disaster. More important and more serious are the misconceptions, for example, in respect of the advisory structure where some groups believe the acceptance of their advice to be near mandatory while others feel aggrieved that a similar, apparently privileged, channel of communication is not open to them. The whole area of joint consultation and the presentation of advice is confused in the minds of many staff.

It is difficult in the course of an informal discussion to question people systematically or closely on such matters as the objectives, organization and machinery of the health service and it is impossible to generalize about how much should be known, since the involvement and influence of staff is not always a function of their particular duties. This is especially so for shop stewards, members of joint consultative committees, members of advisory committees and members of a board. Inevitably, as I shall explain, people were concerned with their immediate difficulties and the fact, as they saw it, that nothing was being done about the issues relevant to them appeared seldom to have been explained in its overall context. This is not a new problem and must reflect to some extent either an omission in the agendas of the joint consultative committees or a flaw in the mechanism by which the staff members of these committees report back to their colleagues.

One of the results is the growing significance of leadership within the various trade union and professional organizations active within the service. In the absence of an acceptable and identifiable mixed team in the immediate working milieu, it is perhaps not surprising that individuals look solely to their fellow workers for moral support. It is only in a few instances that those working in the health service see themselves as members of a team or even a series of teams; it is perhaps unreasonable to expect that this should be the general view but the absence of this unit identity carries far-reaching implications. The reasons for this lack will be discussed later but one of its unforeseen effects seems to have been an increased tendency to separate into discrete professional, craft or trade groupings. Again, it would be wrong to make too much of these comments or to infer that such loyalties need in any way interfere with the working of the health service; my object is merely to point out the fragmentation of interests and the changing basis of loyalties in the absence of a cohesive structure in the working situation. Attempts must be made not just to achieve good communications but to create a common purpose amongst those brought

into contact during the provision of care and services. Whether nurses, doctors
or administrators, either singly or in combination, are given this duty is of less
importance than the fact that it is done.

(c) Conditions of service

Views about conditions of service were strongly held and correlated closely
with how recent and how large a pay rise the particular category of staff had received. Nevertheless, it was the general opinion held by most staff that several
health service jobs are undervalued in terms of monetary return. These points
must be recorded because of the frequency with which they were made, as were
questions about subsidized transport, a local weighting and overtime for part-
time workers. The regulations on these matters are explicit but many of the
arguments presented had considerable substance. Understandably, priority has
been given to safety requirements, patients' amenities and clinical services.
Whether these previous priorities are still in accord with the ultimate overall
provision of a satisfactory service in times of staff shortages is a matter for
consideration. Staff cannot be attracted and retained through local improvements in the terms of service and the only scope for inducement lies in improvements in working conditions and in the provision of recreational, social and
supporting facilities. The difficult questions to answer are whether and to
what extent such measures are justified and what would be the returns from
these investments. There is no doubt that, as employers, boards have an
obligation, beyond mere matters of hygiene and safety, to improve conditions
wherever and whenever possible. This is underway at a pace determined by
other demands and the real issue is whether a higher priority should now be
accorded to this sector.

(d) Understanding of roles

Without doubt the most severe anxiety expressed by staff related to an absence
of identity both with and within the health service. Spontaneous contentions
of being treated as cyphers to be moved or ordered about without explanation
were frequent but when challenged were modified to feelings rather than facts.
Nonetheless, the impersonal insensitive aura is widely felt. When explored,
it is true that particular members of staff are moved at short notice to make
up for unexpected shortages, but a proportion of these individuals know that
they are employed to cover just such contingencies. When explored further,
there is a widespread uncertainty regarding the scope, form and precise nature
of responsibilities within the reorganized health service. This anxiety is real

and obviously cannot be dismissed. It is often difficult for the outsider to understand the origins of the anxiety, for in many cases the duties of posts appear to be identical to those required of the holders before reorganization. Frequently the complaint was made that few people appeared willing to make decisions and that queries were now passed on up the line where previously such problems had been resolved at department or hospital level. It was claimed that the explanation given for such referrals was that the individuals concerned no longer believed or understood that such matters could be determined by their discretion. In some ways this situation is self-perpetuating: the thought is father to the fact and it is but a short stage to the feeling that the organization is unconcerned with the individual. Even more serious are the signs that people are no longer trying to solve problems and the tendency to look critically at other groups as the causes of their difficulties is becoming all too common. People are not facing reality; improvement does not come from an Act of Parliament but from action; if things are in a mess then the sooner everyone tries to sort it out the better.

During the initial discussions it was suggested that the size of the organization, in particular the large central hospital complex, was a major factor in the dissatisfaction being expressed. This possibility was explored but the feelings were present generally throughout the district. A sense of remoteness is largely subjective and the actual loss was focused on the absence (in some cases merely the sense of absence) of a board of management, a medical superintendent, a hospital secretary and a matron. The fact that the term 'matron' was used is significant; when asked, people acknowledged that there is an equivalent grade within the Salmon structure[1] but pointed out that it is the role rather than the post that has disappeared.

It is not the purpose of this paper (nor is the information available) to discuss the reasons for these comments but it is true that the nurses in senior posts within the Salmon structure are themselves aware of a deficiency in that, although their own internal lines of communication are perfectly clear, they are at times uncertain of the other structures and individuals with whom they should be interacting. Comments by ward sisters revealed the need to examine the problem of communications in greater detail and it may be that the question of delegation and the different ways in which the Salmon proposals might be interpreted should be considered at the same time.

Perhaps the most important lesson that has emerged is the fact that size really is not the problem but is merely a convenient butt for criticism; size, of course, creates difficulties but these could be overcome if other problems were first resolved. The real problems arise from the interaction of the attitudes, enthusiasm and expectations of the people concerned. As an oversimplification, the demand is for faster decision-making but if everyone continues to both expect and try to take part in every decision then the health service will grind to a halt. Safeguards exist—the board monitors the executive and the executive monitors its officers; chairmen report to committees and the committee members report to their colleagues. If organizations the size of the health service are to make any progress, then a large part of their business must be based on delegation and accountability.

DISCUSSION OF FINDINGS

Unfortunately, large organizations, particularly with established democratic methods of representation, are slow to respond to changes in the social mood. This predicament has hit the health service severely and the delayed response to the earlier demands for a greater measure of collective staff involvement has thus coincided with the realization that the representatives of the various groups and professions seldom have the delegated authority to negotiate the compromise necessary to achieve action.

It would have been unrealistic to expect that so great a change could have been achieved without some misunderstanding and misdirection and, if these brief generalizations are accepted, then much of the anxiety and uncertainty can be accounted for. First, we need a clear picture of our problems. The board and also the staff must ask questions of themselves, of their work and methods of work, of their relationships and of their images. Our communications have been blocked, partly because the personnel are not all in post, partly because the structures are untried and partly because the people concerned are not fully committed to nor fully understand the changes under way. As a result, people are becoming increasingly uncertain, unconvinced or disillusioned, and this cannot be altered by edict; people are no longer influenced (and certainly not convinced) in this way.

The process by which the staff realize their dependence on others and in turn appreciate the dependence of others on them must be continued. In any large organization problems will always exist but inevitably through time they change. The need is to be aware of their existence and their nature and to recognize the possibility that we are responsible in some part for them. This applies to a board as to any other group of staff and in particular to the relationship of a board to its senior officers and executive groups. There is evidence of a conflict here over whether the latter are expected to administer or manage.

It became clear during the discussions with staff that a forum for airing anxieties and clearing up misunderstandings was both useful and necessary. It also emerged that staff with other duties were not always able to give adequate time for this purpose and more importantly were often thought by the people seeking information not to be able to afford time for such approaches. Being required by undertaking this investigation to find the time and in a sense stand back and observe, we soon became aware of the need to explain one part of the service to another. It is not suggested that the discussions had in any real measure made up for this deficiency but in both the preparation of reports and discussion with staff new uses of existing data have been demonstrated and misconceptions have been corrected. In a sense a need had been found rather than met but at the same time the potential benefits of meeting this need have been partially revealed.

It appears that this by-product of the activities associated with this study should now become a prime function and that a facility should be created specifically to provide information and answer questions. The board takes on so much work now that a central information desk is justified for general matters rather than for the more specific queries which should be answered by those directly responsible. It is likely that most of the queries will be within the competence of those given this duty either to answer directly or to route the enquiry to others possessing the specialist information or responsibility. Examples are the passing of specific queries over wages or salaries to the appropriate finance officer; the answering of general questions on conditions of service, Whitley regulations or the purpose of a particular committee by the staff manning the enquiry station.

Staff suggested appointing a local ombudsman, but from the experience gained during the study the provision of information at an early stage would seem likely to prevent problems and be preferable to a mechanism merely for resolving problems that might more easily have been averted. The staff of the enquiry station would not deal with complaints but would point out to the enquirer the existing mechanisms and appropriate person for dealing with the matter raised. This in itself would be a valuable service.

Once established such a facility could be used in other ways. From the enquiries raised, appropriate topics for study days and in-service education could be suggested or suitable articles proposed for the local health services news sheet. Another important function would be liaison between the advisory and consultative committees and, in conjunction with the executive group, minutes or abstracts of non-confidential meetings could be catalogued and made available to *bona-fide* enquirers. Finally, in association with other sections or departments, position papers or special reports based perhaps on a study day or *ad hoc* meeting might be prepared at the request of the board, executive group or other recognized group within the service.

When described in these terms this new facility has much in common with the National Health Service Centres; indeed, these are a good parallel because the aim would be to provide similar services (information, education, demonstration and reporting) but geared to the more local needs and issues relevant to all the staff of a health board. Again, it is not suggested that this would do away with the need for discussions and meetings between the staff themselves but rather the aim would be to provide first the information, second the opportunities and, third, the guidance to make such meetings effective.

One possibility would be to associate this facility closely with the personnel department as this appears to represent a logical and interesting development of the personnel function.

CONCLUSIONS

It seems that most people no longer believe what is being said or doubt the competence and integrity of other groups—certainly this is what the general behaviour and attitudes imply. If so, then representatives from the groups concerned must state their suspicions and doubts to the people they believe to be at fault. If this is not so then people should clearly indicate perhaps not their satisfaction with the present situation, but certainly their understanding and acceptance of the situation. Confidence will only be restored if staff will talk to each other and have their questions answered. Some people may feel there is already too much talking and to an extent this is true; but most of the talking is within groups and in view of the context and topics understandably has carried a considerable measure of self-interest.

The climate will not improve until we all start exchanging views and understanding the nature of each other's attitudes. We do not have to agree, we may hold private regrets but a continuation of our present positions and attitudes is likely to destroy slowly the very services we are trying to provide.

In addition to these internal stresses the health service is perpetually beset by two other external problems, namely what it is expected to achieve and the finance allowed to attain its goals. The problems are all interrelated and cumulative. First, the various groups within the health service are in no way agreed on their roles, responsibilities and relationships. Without such agreement it is not possible to define goals. Without goals it is not possible to rationalize the use of available resources. Without a demonstrably fair distribution of resources neither the public nor those working in the service are likely to feel confident or committed. Somewhere this cycle must be broken.

Before reorganization it was believed by management that integration would allow the definition of goals and the rationalization of resources—unfortunately, the implications of deteriorating morale were either discounted or not recognized. Now, some 18 months after reorganization, no one is willing to accept or believe the statements or assurances of virtually anyone else. Chairmen of boards, members of executive groups or chairmen of advisory committees who believe otherwise are deceiving themselves.

It may appear that to suggest that the solution lies in discussions between groups of staff is trivial or naive but if people distrust each other there is no other way than to talk it out. At the end, not everyone must be in agreement but a sufficient level of confidence may have been restored for the organization to carry the doubters.

It is possible to translate these generalizations into needs that would be applicable to local situations. First, there should be no further organizational change until a reasonable period of at least a further two years of readjustment has been allowed.

Second, considerable efforts should be made to aid the development of an interface between the consultative and advisory structures. These committees are the only means through which staff can participate in the administration and management of local services. This is not a duty of a board or its officers, but an offer of assistance and concern should be made.

Third, there is urgent need to define responsibilities, duties, channels of communications and procedures for complaints, particularly for supervisory and managerial staff, irrespective of profession. This information might be presented as a set of guidelines (as opposed to directives) indicating the development of job content. All administrators and middle managers have a prime responsibility to stimulate and improve communications. Any activities which achieve this should be part of their job guidelines and because of the overlapping nature of the duties of the various professions it is appropriate, at this stage of integration, to define these new functions in some detail. Lest this seems to be stating the obvious it is opportune to remember that many of the complaints in this study focused on what, it was claimed, had been lost and, therefore, it seems necessary to tell people what they ought to be doing.

Fourth, such guidelines need not be fixed and their updating could well stem from discussions in the joint advisory committees already suggested. Job descriptions framed in this way could also cover the questions of delegation and accountability which are the keys to effective action within the reorganized service. The making of decisions at the correct level of management avoids the growing obstacle, referred to earlier, of everyone expecting to be consulted. The protection or monitor is accountability which, as a result, must be an integral component of delegation. The selection of someone in medicine, nursing and administration whose responsibility would be to foster the exchange of ideas and problems between the various groups providing care and services for patients would be a case in point. Job guidelines should be made widely available and might form the basis of interprofessional seminars or study days organized locally. As I have already indicated, the modification and improvement of problems will only come through discussions between staff; people should be encouraged to ask for information and explanations from each other and from the board. A board's responsibility is, within the resources available, to provide the opportunities.

Fifth, there is no need for extra staff to achieve these communications. The need is to reassess priorities in the light of these comments and accordingly to modify or, if unconvinced, to continue our present activities.

Perhaps I should make a final comment about a likely time scale. Discussions of this nature would take many months and logically must be phased to allow time to deal with the three sets of problems in an appropriate sequence. Initially, staff must sort out their apparent differences and establish equitable and effective communications. Secondly, through these channels, agreement on policies, priorities and programmes must be reached within the services. Finally, once those within the services see a way through the difficulties of resource allocation, a further round of discussions not just with representatives of the board but also with those providing the services must be held to involve the public in agreement over future priorities.

ACKNOWLEDGEMENT

I am most grateful to the study group, staff and members of the Grampian Health Board for their advice and assistance.

Discussion

Bridger: An essential feature is the relationship between the Department and the health boards or the health authorities. Speaking personally, I seriously question the professional wisdom of those who advised on the reorganization of the National Health Service in accepting an assignment to redesign the health service on pseudo-consultative lines while leaving the Department of Health and Social Security outside that system. What are your views of the criteria you are setting up?

Weir: I should mention that I am a member of the health board lest it seem that I am too critical of the boards. It is as a member that I have seen the problems; boards now receive directions from the central Department which commit totally their resources and we are in no position to make real policy decisions. All we do, in a sense, is rubberstamp the recommendations that have come through and our treasurer then tells us how much more development money has been taken away. As one progresses through the various parts of the organization, there is no motive for people to take responsibility. In fairness, part of the problem may be the result of the reorganization which means that people are trying to find what is expected of them and the same difficulties probably exist at the centre as at the periphery. In addition, we have financial problems and development monies have been cut. Perhaps this pre-empting of resources is therefore being exaggerated, but it is unfortunate that it happened at this time because it has taken away the very means by which we could have put some enthusiasm and commitment back into the service.

Baderman: If there is some fundamental difficulty (whether real or imagined) between central authority and a tier or body which looks as impressive as the health board, it is small wonder that the individual feels the most crippling and damaging difficulty, almost to the point of impotence, in his concept of his new role. With all the propaganda and publicity (which I hope was sincere) about enthusiastic individuals being given more chance to play a wider role, to take more responsibilities, why do so many people feel that they have less chance? Central to this may be the difficulties over identity of role, role anxiety, what our responsibilities are and where the direction and the leadership are coming from. The individual who previously thought (maybe misguidedly) that he could do something, not just for his own little empire but perhaps for the greater good, now is convinced that he cannot—and maybe in fact he cannot. Something went wrong.

Roy: When people do not make decisions it is because they doubt their competence to do so. From a clinician's viewpoint, the reorganization has resulted in the 'supercharged Peter Principle':[2] people have risen to the level of their incompetence, and even far above it. This results from the natural desire to receive salary promotion and the reluctance of colleagues to interfere with this promotional 'creep' while it was going on. Some management techniques for fostering confidence seem to misfire for the lack of attention to detail. Staff appraisal is an example when carried out without its function being explained to staff who are already insecure. The prospect of being appraised makes them even more fearful of their superiors—a situation which could hardly be more calculated to disrupt a management structure.

Knox: Dr Weir need not worry about giving away secrets; many of us have expressed concern that guidelines from the Department of Health and Social Security are likely to be more regulatory than advisory and that they would as likely as not cut across initiatives taken by district management teams and area health authorities. The development of effective planning is fraught with difficulties, by no means lessened by the Department's *Guide to Planning in the*

NHS, issued in draft early in 1975, which describes what *should* happen but apart from sketching out configurations of relationships and a set of printed forms—in effect 'bids' for resource allocations—does not give much help in *how* to plan. Health service planning is in its infancy, particularly in the UK. It tends to be thought of simply as a way of assessing problems, weighing their importance, evaluating and selecting appropriate decisions, and then finally recommending action. This view is inaccurate because it is incomplete. As Emery & Trist[3] have pointed out, however technical many of its aspects may be, planning is a *social* process and is, in itself, a political activity. Following Monnet, some French planners have based their practice on a recognition of a simple and fundamental truth: that planning is not so much a programme as a process, and that it is continuous, with phases of formulation, implementation, evaluation and modification which succeed and interact with each other without reaching a final limit.

Goulston: I wonder whether similar problems were encountered when the National Health Service began in 1948. Are they inherent in any new organization? Further, it seems we have fostered a national pastime. The English love cross-word puzzles, they love to consider and discuss problems. Are we not all colluding and playing at an enormously elaborate game while we are wondering which way perhaps we might move forward?

Weir: In 1948, the administration of the health board with which I am associated consisted of five officers; now, it must be about 70. At the beginning, there was fantastic scope to do something and to create services. With reorganization we have a structure which has only to sort itself out. As Dr Knox said, *Guidelines* denied us that scope which was open to our predecessors in 1948. No Machiavellian plot exists; that is just how it looks. With due respect to the Department, it was incompetent to allow different sections to issue these guidelines without putting them together and finding that they represent more than the resources that the boards have available. There are so many directives coming at us that we have no time to recover.

Huntingford: One need high on your list was the establishment of a common purpose. I dispute, however, that we should go about this by putting our own house in order first from within. This would be an introspective way of looking at the problem, because it excludes the people for whom the health service exists. We seem to have lost our sense of purpose for just this reason—all of us as professionals have excluded the people who we are meant to serve. Community health councils should not be the last bodies to join the process; correction from outside is what the health service badly needs.

Weir: I take the point. My anxiety is timing. If we carry the debate outside the health service at this time, I fear that the service will be in real danger of collapse. That might be a good thing, enabling us to start again. My experience of local health councils makes me wary; they are a strange mixture in terms of representation; they do not feel bound by any codes of confidentiality, in that they believe genuinely that their duty is to inform the public—for instance, by prematurely leaking information to the press. Therefore, until we are sorted out, public exposure of our wounds and sores could be dangerous.

Huntingford: Apparently it has only taken a short time to reach the present crisis within the health service, because of reorganization and the socioeconomic situation. But dissatisfaction has been growing for at least a decade. I am not convinced that we need or deserve to buy more time.

Weir: I concede that as a view.

Huntingford: One condition of service that generates dissatisfaction, which does not involve money, hours of work or whether married quarters are provided, is over-elaboration of training for young doctors by the professional leaders. We keep young doctors in subjugation too long, withholding responsibility, so that they become cynical and disillusioned, instead of promoting the development of a sense of responsibility by giving it at a young age. Such dissatisfaction results in demands for alternative compensation in terms of higher salaries.

Hockey: Surely the measure of democratic management with consumer participation and the speed of decision-making have to be inversely correlated? We seem to have to make a choice between full consumer participation on the one hand and rapid decisions on the other. I am sure that we have the worst of all worlds at the moment because we have a sham democracy; we have the structure in the letter but not in the spirit. The tremendous bureaucracy appears on paper to be a marvellous mechanism for consumer participation and democratic government but because of the points you made it is destructive of any kind of participation and gives us nothing.

Weir: This is the root of the problem. People come not as delegates from the groups they represent but as spokesmen, who have to return to their groups to get a mandate before making a decision. Consequently, decisions can be delayed for many months or not made at all. No service can work in that way, but that is the structure we have been given to try to operate.

Beckhard: I sympathize with the doctor or the health worker in this situation who has to decide whether to treat a set of symptoms and make the patient (i.e. the worker in the health service) feel better or whether to go to the fundamental causes, which might be the people in the community or the relationship between them and the system. Further, what are the costs of following either alternative?

At the Sloan School of Medicine, we have been studying how institutions change. One finding is that three states of change exist: what *was* (for instance, before the reorganization of the health service); what *will be* (the reorganized health service in action); and *transition*. Superficially, transition appears like the second state (the health service is officially reorganized), but in reality it is not the new state, rather it forms a bridge between the old and the new. Institutions tend to manage this transition either through the old management system or through the new management system for the new state. What is usually needed is a new and unique management system for this transition state. Dr Weir said, for example, that an information system would be one solution. Our experience in other settings leads us to suggest that a new management system ought to be created. In an area health authority or board, a project manager could be appointed for the transition in designated areas or a group of representatives from the various disciplines or professions could be gathered together as a transition management organization. Unless some such mechanism is created to deal with such a complex change as the reorganization, natural effects such as those you described are inevitable. But one cannot do more than treat the symptoms by dealing with all the things that you mentioned. For example, clarification of job descriptions will neither change the problem nor specify roles, because the emphasis wrongly stresses roles rather than tasks. The problem will be solved when people with different roles look at common vital work to decide what behaviour is appropriate for different roles in different classes of work. We have found that many difficulties originate in dilemmas in the relationships between personnel at different levels of an institution, for example the Department and the area, the area and the workers, the community and the patients. Where this is so, it is at the middle levels rather than the top or bottom of the institution that the problems need to be managed.

Weir: I have noticed that the area executive group has taken on this transitional function, but only by force of circumstance. But the members of the group are now not free to do the jobs that they were appointed to do and inevitably they have taken some authority away from the district officers.

Beckhard: There are several possible management mechanisms: the existing executive group, the hierarchy, a representative group of the constituencies, an *ad hoc* group of natural leaders. It is important to publicize the group that has been chosen to manage the transition as well as the fact that it exists with special and specific functions. The executive group, for instance, may have to take on new responsibilities in addition to its normal management tasks. The different and additional functions of the same group must be made explicit.

Tait: If lack of trust between groups is the problem—and that is the sense of what we are saying—then surely we ought to construct task groups that cut across other professional groups. What are the task groups that make functional sense in the National Health Service? It seems to me that the individual ward in the district general hospital and the group practice are examples of this kind of task-oriented working group. We might have to unscramble some of the administrative machinery we have constructed in order to get these natural functional units to thrive.

Levitt: I find it difficult to see how the solution will be reached when the problem that you identified is perpetuated in your suggested order, Dr Weir. You have been very possessive about information and discussion—as you said, *within* the health service. Surely the consultative bodies, such as local health councils and the local authorities, are 'within' the health service for the purpose of solving the problem, and unless they are brought in closely and early, the problem will be perpetuated.

Weir: More than one road leads to Mecca. With regard to the local health councils, it will be difficult enough to sort out the problems of the health service without bringing in other bodies at this stage.

Levitt: You mentioned the embarrassment caused by local health councils breaking confidentiality. But one should ask why they did it, why they leaked information to the press. Perhaps these councils do not perceive the information in the same way that you do. Is enormous damage done when more people than the members of just one group know about it? Only by questioning such assumptions will one be able to find solutions.

Weir: A subsidiary question is, what has the creation of community health councils as an advisory group that the regional health board must consult done to their planning process and to the way they make proposals? Members of the councils have tended to jump the gun and assume that proposals are plans, hence the confusion. Boards have to fly kites to find out which proposals people prefer but political capital can be made from premature and partial disclosures. This is no way for a health council and health board to operate.

Levitt: In practice, you suggested that groups of staff discuss and find interfaces; how do you do that? What do you tell people when you have got them together? How do you encourage them to talk about what may solve their problems?

Weir: I should like to give the paper I have just presented to administrators, ward maids, consultants, nurses, housemen, porters—a cross-section from the service willing to sit down and discuss it. After that, we could define areas of conflict. Often one group defines its jobs and responsibilities in isolation only to be confronted by another group who claim that they really make the decisions. We must sort these disagreements out amongst ourselves, because if we involve other people at this stage the whole service may collapse.

Levitt: Who are the others? I question your rigid distinction between those within the National Health Service and those outside it.

Arie: We have been working in this field for four years totally unaware that Dr Weir was, too! About three years ago we published similar conclusions about the components of what is called morale but our interest was focused at the micro level rather than the macro level of the National Health Service surveyed by Dr Weir.[4] We were concerned with the tasks that needed to be done by ward staff. Although there have been great developments, particularly since the war, in recognition of the importance of measuring need and of how effectively services meet that need, the 'staff factor'—namely, concern with the meaning of the work for the staff, the ways in which staff are able to do the work and their gratification from it—is still much neglected. May Clarke, a sociologist who was working with us, studied nurses in long-stay wards for old people. Her view of the components of morale was similar to Dr Weir's list, comprising factors such as favourable attitudes towards the organization and sympathy with its goals; sympathy with the peer group; hopefulness and enthusiasm about the work and a feeling that goals can be achieved; satisfaction with the status of the job, the working conditions, the prospects of promotion; satisfactory relations with individual colleagues—in short, 'morale' is a very complex concept. Morale can be high even when people are out of sympathy with the hierarchy; indeed, the tension of dissent can generate morale. Is there a way in which these studies can be more effectively disseminated? Few people seem to be working on such matters; the Department of Health and Social Security supports few studies of what might be called staff morale.

Bridger: I cannot agree that morale is conditional solely on what happens in the hierarchy. Admittedly, morale was high when we were fighting Hitler but after the war the changed situation could not be so easily explained. Morale can also be short-term or long-term. One needs to understand the situation, the context and the conditions at the time.

Weir: We began our project because, with the development of the oil industry in North-East Scotland and the concomitant building of many hotels, many staff (ward maids, porters, catering staff, etc.) left the hospital service. The problem was how to recruit and retain staff. The method used in *Hospitals Communication Project* was no use to us, and instead we used an approach similar to that in the army manual on *Man Management*. We chose the four headings and examined their relevance to our morale because we needed quick solutions. We have to solve the central problem perhaps by discussions between the staff before we can even talk about resources. We are bound by the re-organized system within which we are now operating, short of the revolution, which I fear is too drastic a solution.

Beckhard: To be a devil's advocate, I must point out the danger: many studies have proved that there is practically no correlation between high morale and high productivity. (That finding is common across cultures and segments of society.) If the sole object is high morale, the result will not be effective decision-making—it will not necessarily make the National Health Service function any better. One must concentrate on getting the work done more effectively, on collaboration around work, on allocation of resources and so on. Morale in the system has to be high enough to produce the energy to do the work.

Baderman: Dr Weir, you mentioned commitment; that is an important ingredient but not the same as morale. If commitment is energy for work, I wonder how you measure it, let alone engender or increase it?

Weir: I am reporting only one study out of the five we mounted. We considered four other issues that we thought might improve the local service.

References

1 MINISTRY OF HEALTH, SCOTTISH HOME AND HEALTH DEPARTMENT (1966) *The Salmon Report of the Committee on Senior Nursing Structure*, HMSO, London
2 PETER, L.J. & HULL, R. (1969) *The Peter Principle: Why Thing Always Go Wrong*, Morrow, New York
3 EMERY, F. & TRIST, E. (1973) From planning towards the surrender of power, in *Towards a Social Ecology*, Plenum, London and New York
4 ARIE, T. (1972) Aspects of the Goodmayes Service, in *Approaches to Action* (a symposium on Services for the Mentally Ill and Handicapped) (McLachlan, G., ed.), Oxford University Press (for Nuffield Provincial Hospitals Trust), London

The response of the hospital doctor to the health requirements of a changing society

DOUGLAS ROY

Department of Surgery, The Queen's University of Belfast

Abstract Before the advent of the National Health Service in 1948 most hospital doctors were in close contact with the primary care of, at least, a section of the community both by their continuing close contacts with general practitioners and as a result of often having spent some part of their careers as general practitioners. Since 1948 this awareness of the health aspirations of the community has weakened as a result of advances in the care of disease which have made the hospital doctor increasingly dependent on sophisticated facilities and, thus, focused his attention on hospital care rather than on the community.

Hospital staff must re-establish their link with primary care and must perceive clearly the ways in which they contribute to the health of their community. They must be conscious of the proportion of available resources that are used in hospital and be prepared to regulate demands so that there is equality in the distribution of resources in the health field. Hospitals are not only expensive but have become extravagant; it is the responsibility of the hospital doctor to curb extravagance. If private practice is to continue, it must be integrated into the health service, not excluded from it.

Finally, the patient must be recognized as a member of a family and of a community that is both curious and concerned about health. The hospital doctor must communicate with patience, understanding and clarity. In this relationship he also has a part to play in health education and prevention of disease. He must remove the mystery from his art and enter into useful discussions with government and community.

There is a widespread feeling, expressed both in the lay and the medical press, that the staffs of our hospitals have become remote from the wishes of the community about its health. The recent disastrous reorganization of the health service was an attempt to redress the balance between hospital and community services but there is little evidence so far that they are coming together. In retrospect it becomes obvious that we have deceived ourselves, and still do so, into thinking that shuffling an administrative structure will change attitudes; in practice, it has led to confrontation and a resistance to change. If attitudes are to respond to changes in the wishes of the community (however ill-expressed they may be) and to diminishing resources, the changes must be generated by the physicians themselves in dialogue with other members of the community. When one listens to statements from the British Medical Association and other professional bodies, one can be pessimistic about the chances that they have the will, the insight or the intelligence to undertake this responsibility. There is, however, a substantial minority that is aware of the problems and would be able to produce solutions, provided that they are encouraged to do so by the support of their colleagues and of the government.

Many doctors do not think about the problems of our society because it has never occurred to them that they have a responsibility to do so; they were certainly not taught to do so by those clinicians they usually admired as students. The study of social medicine was (and still is, sometimes) ridiculed by clinicians teaching students in hospitals.

Before the advent of the health service in 1948 the medical profession had not long emerged from a struggle to establish itself and to formalize the standards of conduct that this implied. The central point of this code of conduct was that the patient's interests were paramount. A patient was someone who had sought out the doctor and asked for his care or who had been admitted to one of his beds in a hospital. The hospital doctor was not remote from the community. He had, after all, often spent part of his early career in general practice and continued to be in close contact with general practitioners on whom he depended for most of his income. He visited the homes of patients with the general practitioner, and a harmonious (and rewarding) relationship existed between them which benefited the patient. Unfortunately, it only embraced a section of the community and certainly excluded the poorer families who often depended on a general practitioner with a 'lock-up' shop as his consulting room and on the charity of voluntary hospitals or the meagre facilities of a local authority hospital. In those days, the hospital doctor was certainly responsive to the needs of the families he knew but only a few concerned themselves with the large urban populations in the poorer social classes. The result was that the middle and upper classes and rural population were well and economically cared for in both private and public hospitals while some of the poorer urban population received inadequate and often unfeeling care.

Many, if not most, hospital doctors have not yet realized that one implication of a National Health Service is the change in definition of the word patient and thus the change in scope of their responsibility. The patient is no longer only the person in the consulting room or hospital bed but everyone who might now or later require the skills that the doctor or his colleagues possess. The doctor must, therefore, discharge his responsibility to the patient he has not yet seen as well as to the ones he sees now. The importance of this new concept becomes increasingly clear as advances in medical technology provide the hospital with more complicated and expensive methods of treating disease, especially as the gain in benefit may not always be proportional to the increase in the cost. Under the older concept the doctor must fight for everything the patient needs even to live one extra day and, if all were equally good (or fair) fighters, then a balance would eventually be struck that would perhaps be equitable. Unfortunately, some are better (or less scrupulous) fighters than others so that the end result is an uneven distribution of resources within the hospital service. Furthermore, the hospital doctor generally wins any fight with other sections of the health service.

Advances in medical technology have another effect. They are so complex and fascinating that the hospital doctor resists being distracted from them by the problems of apportionment of resources which may be more important to his patients. A good surgeon finds it difficult to see why he should have responsibilities other than to see that his patients recover quickly and are restored to good health. It is so self-evident that he is doing 'a good job'. What more should be asked of him? He does not usually realize that his reputation and, often, formidable appearance guarantee him the equipment and facilities that will be denied the geriatrician. Nevertheless, it should not be for administrators to force priorities on doctors; it would be better if doctors were to decide these themselves on the basis of facts supplied by the administration. Administration should be efficient and unobtrusive, and must foster the dialogue between doctor and community. This dialogue must not be obstructed by an inappropriate administrative structure.

Private practice now forms a small part of the activities of hospital doctors and its rewards are the icing on the cake rather than the cake itself. It leads to only superficial contacts with a small section of the community. In England and Wales only 50% of consultants are engaged in private practice; in Scotland and Northern Ireland the proportion is less. Domiciliary consultations form the main contact with the general practitioner, but even this has gone amiss: it is no secret that often these consultations become just a means of by-passing a waiting list; sometimes the general practitioner is not even present when the patient is seen. Attempts to include hospital doctors in the new health centres have not been easy. At Livingstone (New Town) joint appointments between hospital and general practice were partially successful, but the general practitioner with a hospital appointment found that he was more a registrar than a consultant and unlikely to influence events in hospital. There has, therefore, been little in the past 30 years to direct any portion of the interest of hospital doctors towards an understanding of the general needs and aspirations of the community. This situation has been made worse in the past few years by the doctors' apprehension that inflation and social change are diminishing their status and prosperity in relation to other sections of the community so that, understandably, their concern is turned inwards and they have become yet another section of the community fighting for what they believe to be their rights and are unconcerned about the community as a whole. It has become a very poor climate for change.

The one good thing about the recent reorganization was the attempt to integrate hospital and other community services (although—except in Northern Ireland—the personal social services were regrettably excluded) and this must be the basis on which the links with primary care are re-established. General practitioners should be allowed access to the investigative and therapeutic facilities of the hospital; some might be unable to use them but this is because they have not been allowed to do so and have, therefore, lost an ability they once had. The use of such facilities with the help and advice of the consultants could become an enduring link bringing benefits to patients and doctors and reducing the need to admit patients to hospital. Community hospitals must be developed, run by general practitioners with consultants visiting as often as necessary. There are many small hospitals which struggle to maintain acute medical and surgical units but whose role should be that of a community hospital. Consultants should still visit them and see outpatients and referred patients even though acute beds would be in the regional hospital. Consultants should also have commitments to visit health centres and, by coming to know the general practitioners, would become sensitive to their needs and problems and appreciate their generalist abilities. Every community should have consultant hospital doctors to share the responsibility for providing the community with the best medical care possible. The hospital doctor must cease to believe that his responsibilities are confined to the place where he has his beds.

The influence of private consulting practice cannot be ignored. The monumental folly of excluding it from the health service and thus further distracting the attention of consultants from their responsibilities to the community is only matched by the stubborn idiocy of the representatives of the consultants who seem to imagine that the present system is above reproach and should be retained at all costs for ever. There is not a single original idea to be found on either side.

It has been agreed that private practice should continue. Should it not then be integrated into the health service and controlled in the interests of both public and private patients? Perhaps it is naive to suggest that this could easily be achieved in the following way:

(1) by making private beds available in all teaching, reference and district hospitals;

(2) by having a common waiting list for public and private patients;

(3) by charging the patient the cost of his accommodation and care, less his basic entitlement in a public ward, but plus a surcharge for the benefit of the hospital group (including staff facilities);

(4) by the hospital charging all consultant fees to the patient and paying them to the consultant less a deduction which would be retained for the benefit of the hospital and its staff—there should be an agreed scale of fees;

(5) by making consultants 'geographically full time' and, therefore, available at all times for the care of the patients in that hospital as well as for teaching, research, etc.

If this led to an increase in private practice, as it probably would, it would be private practice within the context of total health care and would inevitably increase again the contacts between consultant and general practitioner to their mutual benefit. The rise of exclusive private hospitals must be resisted; the only alternative and logical policy is to ban private practice altogether.

Hospitals are expensive places. At a time when resources are diminishing, it is inevitable that the money available for the development of hospitals will be restricted in the interests of other aspects of health care. It is better that these economies are formulated by hospital doctors rather than imposed by authority. One despairs of consultants being able to do this but it would certainly be worth the effort to try to persuade them to do so. Hospitals are also extravagant and it is disturbing to see the casual waste of equipment and facilities that occurs in every hospital every day. Self-discipline is required and it should not be considered beneath the dignity of a consultant to be informed of his drug bill in relation to that of his colleagues so that he can exert a degree of control over the cost of the service he provides.

Few consultants believe that they have a function to perform in preventive medicine and health education. They are, however, in a unique position to do both. As they are seen to be expert at curing disease, people will easily believe that they must also know how to prevent and avoid disease. Nobody should ever treat disease without considering how it could be prevented. Patients today are better informed and more curious than ever before; it is the doctor's duty to satisfy these aspirations with patience, understanding and clarity. Medical technology must be, as Mahler[1] says, 'demystified' so that the doctors can join in a reasonable dialogue with government and community.

The education of the doctor is the source of some of his attitudes but medical students acquire much of their motivation and attitudes from the society in which they live. Society probably gets the doctors it deserves! Nevertheless, the medical schools have considerable opportunities to influence attitudes towards the concept that the health of this country is the concern of everyone. In the past 20 years, although departments of community health have expanded in all medical schools, their influence has been slight. This is because the clinical consultants are still the main teachers and, in general, their attitudes remain unchanged. The community aspects of surgery, medicine, paediatrics or obstetrics should be taught by the consultants in these disciplines. Furthermore, they must endorse the views of their non-clinical colleagues who teach the wider aspects of social medicine. They might even speak to them occasionally!

All this is concerned with developed countries. It is even more true and urgent for developing countries where hospital doctors crowd into the urban areas and, except for a few dedicated ones, are unconcerned about the mass of the population. They sense that their contribution to the health of the nation is a minor one and are afraid that they will lose their status. If they could open up their attitudes and talk realistically about their contribution they would find that they were an important element in health care. They must be specialists for communities rather than specialists in hospitals.

The hospital doctor must turn again to the world outside the hospital. He must restore his links with primary care; he must set his hospital into a scheme of things with no over-riding priorities. He must learn to judge priorities and see himself as being involved in preventive medicine and health education. Above all he must teach others that all this is so.

Discussion

Huntingford: The selection of medical students should ensure that in future the profession is a cross-section of society, which it neither has been nor is but needs to be if society is to get the doctors that it deserves.

Roy: We probably get what we deserve. Today people are rushing after security (e.g. academic qualifications), so new medical students are well qualified and most are looking for a secure job. I should be delighted if the science faculties again attracted *la crème de la crème*. If so, medicine would attract a much wider scatter of abilities. It is society that is imposing this pattern. Can we interfere with the process?

Huntingford: We could relax the academic requirements for entry to medical schools, but we do not.

Bridger: This happens in many developing countries, too.

Abercrombie: In the present state of our knowledge, teaching is more important than selection: we get the doctors we teach. Studying at a medical school is such a socializing experience that it makes nonsense of any idea of getting a representative cross-section of society—as soon as students cross the threshold of a medical school they become alike socially.

Roberts: Dr Roy, you suggested that until recently the individual patient has been sacrosanct but now the actions of the hospital doctor (in respect of any one patient) must also take into account a consideration of the needs of those patients who are on his waiting list, of his colleagues' patients (inpatients and outpatients), and indeed of the whole population of the area health authority. What does this imply for the management of a patient, such as a child with spina bifida, a patient with chronic renal failure, or a 70-year-old man with no family who is living alone and is admitted to hospital with bronchopneumonia?

Roy: In our society, we are not, I hope, looking for uniformity; we do not claim one method alone is correct for treating a child with spina bifida. In the past we have made our decisions about these patients without thinking of the wider implication for the family and the community. When a doctor considers all aspects of such a patient and then decides on a certain course of action, that is fine; we expect different views. In the past, clinicians have tended to give priority to the maximum prolongation of life (of any quality) irrespective of the effect on other people in the family and community.

Roberts: You suggested that the doctor can educate patients in the community about prevention. I agree, naturally, but surely what matters is how much time he spends educating and how much time he spends treating. If the primary concern of a doctor is the health of the community with regard to one disease then perhaps he should give up clinical medicine altogether and become 'first an educator, second an administrator, and third a clinician'.[2] I am concerned that the acceptance of the idea that all clinicians should also do some preventive medicine may introduce a certain complacency into the judgement of the relative benefits of each.

Roy: Many hospital doctors are obliged to and want to both treat disease and teach students. Those who go to developing countries to do this come to realize that the only practical way they could reduce the load of disease is to extend their reach outside the hospital both in a curative and a preventive role. Once a doctor does this he must also participate in the education of other health workers and the people.

Elliott: The obligation of the clinician in many developing countries to practise preventive as well as therapeutic medicine is not constrained by the need for privacy in the doctor/patient relationship which we demand. Morley makes this point about learning by overhearing in several of his writings.[3, 4] In his original under-five's clinic in Nigeria, the mother and the child were examined and advised with all the other mothers looking on. This approach gives a great opportunity for providing health education at the same time as dealing with immediate problems. Similarly, the traditional Chinese practitioners in Taiwan[5] practise in only the one room and the whole group listens to and takes part in the discussions of the patient's symptoms and the advice that is being given. We cannot do that in our society and it is an opportunity we lose. Could our culture ever change sufficiently to accept this?

Bridger: It often happens *ad hoc* in waiting rooms!

Guz: I must disagree with Dr Roy about his attack on the concept of the individual patient being sacrosanct. This is the most contentious issue that has so far been raised. When the individual patient ceases to be sacrosanct, the whole structure of what a doctor does changes. This needs debate, but nobody can take part in that debate until they have been ill themselves. To me the individual patient is sacrosanct and I shall shout as loudly as possible to get what is needed for that patient. The point that you did not make is that doctors often push their claims in the hospital to boost their egos; the person who shouts loudest often gets most. One can draw a clear-cut distinction between what is best for the patient and what is best for the ego of the doctor. That I condemn.

Roy: The idea of the patient being sacrosanct has already been questioned. One problem in the National Health Service is inequality of care and that means that some patients are more sacrosanct than others.

Guz: Presumably this situation arose because people did not shout loud enough in the areas that received less resources.

Roy: I am not arguing against the sanctity of the patient's welfare. I am redefining the term 'patient' to include all those who are or may be in our care in the future.

Levitt: Isn't this issue of the sacrosanctity of the patient a red herring? If doctors respect the individuals who need their help, one avoids this false argument.

Tait: The trend you described, Dr Roy, towards the enclosure of the hospital doctor in the UK within the hospital is unique amongst most medical care systems. During the 19th century the specialist became partially divorced from primary care. The National Health Service made this divorce absolute; it made it impossible for him to maintain any kind of contact with primary care. Perhaps one reason why the consultant values private practice is that it still contains an element of this primary and continuing medical care.

Roy: For that reason I suggested that we must think carefully about private practice before excluding it from the National Health Service. All these contacts would be regenerated by appointing a hospital doctor to an area, a community, rather than to a hospital. For instance, the closure of a surgical unit in a small town causes great opposition and concern—surgery has to be done at a bigger hospital some distance away. Why shouldn't the small town still have a surgeon? He will operate in the larger unit but he is still the surgeon for that small town, and it is his responsibility to see that it gets the surgical service it needs. That is a meaningful contact.

Baderman: As one of the 'will-o'-the-wisps' who slipped through Dr Abercrombie's selection net some years ago, I know what she means about student selection. Just as thinking about perfect student selection may be a fallacy, the sanctity of the individual patient in absolute terms is a myth, too. Any decision about a patient is a management decision: one is making choices which influence other patients. The difficulties that we are now experiencing are, at least in part, due to the fact that such painful processes as making choices have come out into the open: one must consider the district, the waiting list etc. Doctors have been doing that all the time, reluctantly, unwillingly or even subconsciously. Those who have not been doing it because they shouted loudest must take some responsibility, however unwillingly, for inequalities in the distribution of resources. Of course, the sanctity of the patient is an important concept in a purely clinical phase of the whole performance, but that is only one phase, one aspect of a doctor's life, it is not a reality for much of the time.

Arie: Weed[6] reminded us that no consideration of the needs of all the people means poorer care for most of the people. Tudor Hart[7] made a proposal which has to do with the relative influence of selection of medical students compared with the influence of what we do to them. I go along with Dr Abercrombie in believing that selection is not the answer, even though there is self-evident justice in taking a more equitable spread of students who apply for medicine. Students are all right when they begin studying—it is what we do to them that goes wrong. But a good case does exist for looking at other sources of recruitment. Tudor Hart's suggestion was that 20% of the intake into medical schools should be from health service personnel—nurses, technicians, social workers. The fruits of this would be two-fold: first, it would bring into medicine people of a different outlook who had chosen to enter medicine in their maturity and, second (and overwhelmingly important), it would begin to demystify and de-elitize medicine by helping it to become a potential career for any health worker rather than an encapsulated part of health services, closed and self-contained. Doctors, as Dr Roy was saying, have multiple roles of which a principal one is that of teacher. Doctors are rarely taught to assess their role or to question the social function of medicine. Doctors are taught medical techniques, but our training does not encourage us to think about the social implications of doctor-patient transactions. A great deficit in medical education is that it does not attempt to give doctors insight into what medical work means in society.

Gollan: The re-establishment of contact between hospital and the primary care team was discussed by the general practice units in the Kentish Town Health Centre before we moved into new premises in 1973. The centre consists of two practices and it was suggested to the community hospital that we should have attachment from the hospital to the general practice units (rather than the general practitioners going to the hospital, although some do just that) and it was agreed (within the terms of the restructured Health Service and with the agreement of the hospital consultants) that we should have two meetings a month between the general practice teams (health visitors, nurses, students from all disciplines, social workers, doctors) and consultants. Also, while there, the consultant would see three or four patients who had been referred directly from the surgery to see a specialist. That arrangement itself lifted an enormous amount of fear and worry, from mothers and children particularly. A paediatrician and gynaecologist come once a month, and a psychiatrist comes every week and sees three patients. The specialist then discusses with the team the patients he has seen, questions of drug therapy, or anything else that may arise.

We are fortunate that we are near a community hospital; I realize that this arrangement might not be feasible in other areas, but it has been enormously valuable to us in the general practice units and I believe also to the consultants.

Russell: Studies of the devolution of specialist services to health centres have shown not only that the number of referrals to specialists is reduced but also that fewer patients fail to attend when the specialist clinic is held in a health centre.

With regard to the role of hospital doctor, it is difficult to consider all hospital doctors in the same context, because the variety of specialties regulates the extent to which hospital-based doctors can work in the community. Among the highly specialized groups within general medicine a tendency in the opposite direction is evident, which is represented by such statements as 'the job of the specialist as defined in the National Health Service is to give the general practitioner specialized diagnostic and therapeutic advice and, on occasions, to treat; he should, therefore, hand the patient back to the general practitioner as soon as possible, and reduce the amount of clinical supervision in a hospital'. One should not generalize about the hospital doctor.

Roy: I agree; one way of discharging one's duties to the community is to see that the patient is returned to the care of the general practitioner as soon as possible, provided that the contact between hospital doctor and general practitioner is maintained.

Levitt: If about half the consultants in England and Wales (and fewer in Scotland and Northern Ireland) undertake private practice how realistic is your suggestion that private practice should be encouraged? Do your figures for the regions indicate how much private practice doctors want to do or do more consultants want to have private practice but are prevented for various reasons?

Roy: The explanation is simple: there are short waiting lists in Scotland and Northern Ireland—the proportion of consultants to population is higher than in the other regions. Certainly, in Glasgow and in Belfast, few general surgical departments have a waiting list longer than eight weeks. The main impetus at the moment for private practice is the length of the waiting lists. I am suggesting a complete change in the pattern of private practice, so that when a patient's name reaches the top of the list he can choose the clinician or the extra facilities if he so wishes. This would lead to a further beneficial effect. If a hospital had a long waiting list onto which the private patients were being placed, consultants would have a vested interest in making sure it became a short waiting list.

Carter: I greatly favour increased contact between hospital doctors and general practitioners but I am worried about some of the inherent practical problems. Some of the difficulties are pointed out by Hicks:[8] 'For example, in the hospital or hospitals serving a population of 250 000 people there will be, say, somewhere between 40 and 50 consultants. At the same time there will be about 100 general practitioners serving this population at the primary level. Somehow or other each of the 100 general practitioners has to establish good communication with each of the 40 to 50 consultants, each of whom at some time or other during the year may be attending to one or more of his patients. In the reverse direction, each of the 40 to 50 consultants will be attending to patients of each of the 100 general practitioners. It is impossible to manage efficiently a communication system of this kind of complexity on an 'old boy' basis. To make it manageable and reasonably efficient from the point of view of clarity and promptness of the messages that should be passing to and from then a degree of standardisation of messages and request and reporting content is essential .... So far as I know we are a long way from having attempted to get such orderliness into the system'. I doubt whether the system will be able to operate on such a basis, except possibly on a small scale, of which the Kentish Town Health Centre cited earlier may be an example; for a whole health district, it would be impossible to operate.

Gollan: I do not agree with the suggestion that putting private beds alongside public beds would solve the problem of private beds. Considerable evidence shows that many people become private patients in order to jump the queue (see, for example, Mencher,[9] p. 37). A common waiting list would remove much of the justification for private beds. One of the things that most angers many people about private beds in National Health Service hospitals is the sight of two standards side by side.

Roy: Are you arguing for the abolition of private practice?

Gollan: Yes.

Roy: This is a tenable view but neither of the main political parties in this country has suggested it. If we do not abolish private practice, it would be disastrous to force it to become a separate service; it must be included in the National Health Service. I was making certain proposals (which are obviously open to debate) for doing this. Nobody gets indignant about the coexistence of first and second class railway carriages. If, shall we say, a little of the 'gravy' permeated other sections of the hospital service apart from the doctors and if it became accepted that all hospitals had private beds, whether in a separate block or in a modern ward which contained single bed-units, then over the years the steam would go out of the situation: people would cease to buy private treatment in order to skip waiting lists but, if they were provided with facilities (e.g. a phone, television, as much visiting as they liked) and were able to choose their surgeon (if they so desired), there is no reason why they should not be allowed to pay for them. If the Government has its way, there will be glossy new private hospitals in major cities, where the consultants will make a fortune, whereas the consultants in the other towns will have no option but to be full-time NHS workers. The disparity between the rewards for a hospital doctor in the average provincial town and those in the big cities will be enormous. This seems to be the antithesis of socialism.

Weir: An interesting example of misunderstanding about private practice arose during the last confrontation when, locally, medical staff met the unions. For two hours discussion ranged aimlessly until it was discovered that people were using different definitions of private practice. Misunderstandings were considerable: for instance, one group believed that surgeons could receive fees for operating on patients occupying public beds. Once the system was explained all the heat in the local argument vanished and the system of rationing of resources was agreed. Admittedly, one group was travelling first class, but that was acceptable in the interim. I must emphasize that often such arguments arise out of misunderstandings about how the system operates.

Abercrombie: The essence of man is that he is a social animal; we do not exist as individuals isolated from each other. The notion of the doctor dealing with a single patient in isolation relates very much to the parent–child relationship in which, at a certain time, the one-to-one relationship is important. It is ridiculous, however, to imagine treating a child with spina bifida as though he had neither a mother who could look after him nor a family which might be suffering from the effects of 'hyperpaedophilia'.[10] Equally, the doctor is not an individual channelling the effect of his treatment into one person and being able to cure that person in isolation. Dr Elliott's point about practising medicine in public is important and I am not so pessimistic as she seems to be about the possibility of similar things happening here, especially when one considers how even General Franco's illnesses were not his own: the list of the things he was suffering from was everybody's business. This could not have happened 10 years ago. Similarly the widely broadcast fact that two prominent ladies in the USA were operated on for breast cancer was of considerable educational importance. Inadvertently the doctor may do several things (that may or may not be under his control) that express his general attitude; if he believes that he has an important function in educating, he will behave differently even as he operates or writes a prescription, than if he believes that that is his only function. An interesting educational experiment, which extended the therapeutic abilities of the doctor (if one does not regard the doctor as an individual but as part of a network), is Skynner's work with delinquent children.[11] With his team he visited the school from which delinquent children had attended at regular intervals and talked with the staff about their immediate problems and therapeutic procedures. The rate of referral of delinquent children dropped. These children were not individuals outside the community, nor was Skynner an individual doctor shut up in the clinic—he was working in the social matrix. If doctors understood more about these effects, the question of whether their energies be put into teaching rather than into treatment would not arise, for these would be combined.

Tait: In considering the division between clinical and preventive medicine that Dr Roy talked about, we should not get too despondent about the lack of time for preventive medicine. Every clinical moment is potentially useful for converting the patient into an educator both for himself and for others. Problem-orientated records remind me that within my management plans I have diagnostic and treatment plans but also plans for the education of the patient. Every consultation offers a chance to teach a patient how to prevent disease.

Bridger: I initiated the idea of treating the whole hospital as a therapeutic community during World War II at Northfield Hospital, Birmingham. It was based on the notion that a combination of clinical and educational aspects was essential but not just in separate or more limited forms. The patients were most important in a wider consideration of educational development and in the administration as well as in the treatment.

Weir: In this argument over the sanctity of the patient a false difference in terms of treatment of an individual patient and the group seems to be polarizing. Obviously, within the resources available, the clinician shouts once he has determined what an individual patient needs. The apparent issue was that once a group of patients had been defined how far was shouting for further resources for them justified? An excellent example of this was the study of anaesthetic services in hospitals in London, Northampton and Liverpool.[12] The anaesthetists classified all patients who needed their services and focused on the group who required almost instant care. One way of dealing with this was to have an anaesthetist immediately available at all times. They calculated the resources needed for this or for delays of, say, two minutes, five minutes, and so on and concluded that if one were to have a sufficient number of anaesthetists to deal immediately with all situations, nearly all the resources of the National Health Service would be swallowed up in providing anaesthetists. In the event they proposed a scheme whereby the people on call did not necessarily have a full training in anaesthetics but knew how to deal with specific emergencies. I take it that Dr Roy is suggesting that within the resources available there will be no question but that the individual doctor may determine what is needed for that case.

References

[1] MAHLER, H. (1975) Health—a demystification of medical technology. *Lancet 2*, 829–833
[2] KING, M. (1966) in *Medical Care in Developing Countries*, Oxford University Press, London
[3] MORLEY, D. (1966) The under-fives clinic, in *Medical Care in Developing Countries* (King, M.H., ed.), Oxford University Press, London
[4] MORLEY, D. (1973) *Paediatric Priorities in the Developing World*, Butterworths, London
[5] KLEINMAN, A. (1976) The cultural construction of clinical reality: comparisons of practitioner–patient interactions in Taiwan, in *Implications for Health Care of the Cross-Cultural Study of Health, Illness, and Healing* (Harvard Seminar), in press
[6] WEED, L. (1971) Quality control and the medical record. *Archives of Internal Medicine 127*, 101
[7] HART, J.T. (1974) Proposals for assisted entry to medical schools for health workers as mature students. *Lancet 2*, 1191
[8] HICKS, D. (1976) *Primary Health Care: A Review*, HMSO, London, in press
[9] MENCHER, S. (1967) *Private Practice in Britain*, Occasional Papers on Social Administration No. 24, Bell, London
[10] OUNSTEAD, C., LINDSAY, J. & NORMAN, R. (1966) Biological factors in temporal lobe epilepsy. *Clinics in Developmental Medicine 22*, 119–121
[11] SKYNNER, A.C.R. (1974) An experiment in group consultation with the staff of a comprehensive school. *Group Process 6*, 99–114
[12] TAYLOR, T.H., JENNINGS, A.M.C., NIGHTINGALE, D.A., BARBER, B., LEWERS, D., STYLES, M. & MAGUER, J. (1969) A study of anaesthetic emergency work. *British Journal of Anaesthesiology 41*, 70–83

The place of academic research

A. GUZ

Department of Medicine, Charing Cross Hospital Medical School, London

Abstract The medically qualified academic research worker under university aegis but within the National Health Service has recently been subjected to frightening forces. His traditional role of being allowed and financed to do what he wants is questioned in an age of economic crisis and of concern about how to spend limited resources. The call for 'relevance' in academic research makes sense when looked at from society's viewpoint but nonsense when looked at from the research worker's viewpoint.

Recent personal experience has generated a proposal for the resolution, in part, of these conflicting claims; namely, the university hospital. Unless academic research continues to flourish within our present framework, the quality of the practitioners of medicine and paramedical subjects will drop slowly over the next 20 years as the spirit of enquiry dies!

Rightly or wrongly, I feel that I should lay my head on the chopping block for execution. I represent a discipline that has seen a dark cloud recently cover it and that is being asked, 'Do you really merit existence?' It is, therefore, in a spirit of some humility that I should like to describe a little about what we are and what our ethos is.

First, the Oxford English Dictionary defines the term 'academic' in its *modern* setting as 'not leading to a decision' or 'unpractical'. This is to be contrasted with the usage at the end of the 16th century when the term was defined as 'of the school or philosophy of Plato, sceptical, scholarly'. I am sure that this change in meaning reflects some of the troubles that our group is in. In an age of financial squeeze, that which is 'unpractical' is regarded as 'unnecessary'.

Secondly, I shall briefly describe how academic research is organized and then what we, academic research workers, try to do. The main stimulus to the establishment of university departments of medicine came as a result of the visit of the American microbiologist Abraham Flexner[1] to this country in 1912.

His report on the state of medical education advocated the establishment of university nidi in clinical departments. These, he thought, would gradually improve the scientific quality of the medicine practised throughout the hospital and community. Over the next 50 years (!) Flexner's recommendations were more or less implemented. The departments established vary enormously in size, ranging from the 'one-man show' right up to large 'empires'. In all departments, the staff care for patients, teach students, and do research in their subjects. All the departments are heavily dependent on non-university money for the salaries for many of their posts and also for research support.

For the sake of completeness, I should mention that academic clinical research also functions in Medical Research Council units, groups or establishments. These may or may not be associated with hospitals, universities or both.

One may ask whether an individual in a university clinical department can practise medicine, teach students, and advance the subject by academic research. The stresses of attempting to do this are now greater than ever. Nevertheless, it can probably still be done, provided that these departments can resist the current strident call by the districts in which their hospitals exist for *more and more* service to patients. Since patient care must come first, it can, if in sufficient amount, destroy both teaching and research. On the other hand, doing clinical research and teaching in a clinical vacuum may not be particularly rewarding. The problem in a university clinical department is that of striking a balance. One of the best ways of achieving a balance is to have as many clinicians as possible within a department so that, *for each individual*, the amount of time spent in clinical practice and teaching can be kept under some control.

I have time to deal only with three criticisms of what we do.

(1) INHIBITION OF COMPASSION AND UNNECESSARY TESTING

Platt[2] has suggested that, in trying to understand the nature of the disease affecting an individual patient, the university staff investigate so as to provide themselves with occupational therapy! Furthermore, he suggests that the scientific approach may inhibit compassion and insight into the mind and problems of the whole patient. This type of attack has been echoed in other quarters. All I can say about the second accusation is that it is just not true; I doubt if any university clinical department fosters the inhibition of compassion or is not conscious of the profound ethical dilemmas that beset us in both patient care and clinical research. As for the first accusation, Platt may merely be saying that a lot of research needs to be done on which of our tests give us the best discrimination and understanding in any particular disease presentation. This type of accusation often finds expression in the less rigorously formulated idea that we are 'bad clinicians'. It has never been clear to me what this means, but the gibe has often been heard. In general, we have reacted to it by redoubling efforts to provide the highest standards of care; the gibe has acted as a perfect function of forcing one to improve oneself!

(2) LACK OF INTEREST IN PREVENTIVE MEDICINE

We are accused of focusing on the understanding of a disease and its therapy to the detriment of studying its prevention. Rosenheim[3] has opined that 'If, for the next 20 years no further research were to be carried out, if there were a moratorium on research, the application of what is already known, of what has already been discovered, would result in widespread improvement in health'. In this symposium, people have spoken of the preventive art as being something separate from the therapeutic art. I find it difficult to believe that the subject of preventive medicine can flourish in the absence of an *understanding* of disease and an understanding of disease means the use of scientific methods. After all, the prevention of poliomyelitis first needed the virus to be grown; the prevention of phenylketonuria first needed an understanding of the role of phenylalanine in the development of the brain; the prevention of post-operative pulmonary embolism needed an understanding of the use and actions of heparin at all dose levels. These are partial or complete success stories.

A rigorously scientific study of the effects of smoking and raised arterial pressure was first needed before we could even talk about prevention in these areas. In my view, the job of academic clinical researchers is to understand and to teach in relation to preventive medicine. Implementation of many of our deductions may not even be a job for doctors. If the superbly trained health visitors we have been hearing about would accept a new role, then I am sure they would have a much greater impact in preventive medicine than could be achieved by any group of doctors. If they could use what is already known about smoking and hypertension then we should see real preventive medicine implemented and affecting a large section of the adult population.

Why should it be thought that university clinical departments need to focus their attention on *implementation* of preventive medicine?

(3) THE BASIC DISCIPLINES THAT WE USE

Doctors in university clinical departments are applied scientists who bring to bear the traditional disciplines of physics, chemistry, biology, anatomy, physiology and biochemistry into the clinical research arena. This results in the conventional situation of biological mechanisms in health and disease being studied in traditional scientific laboratories. The accusation against us is that we neglect vast areas, such as:

(1) *clinical strategy*, which includes the strategy of the 'follow-up', the strategy of screening, the informed use of tests based on their diagnostic value, and the risks of diagnostic technology;

(2) *health services research*, which includes the relationship between the provider (doctor, nurse, etc.), the health care system, and the patient;

(3) *health policy*, which includes the relationship between ethics, medicine and law.

Here I feel on the defensive, because the accusations ring true. The problem is that in all these areas there is no well-established principle of creative research and people tend to shy away from areas where this holds true. The basic disciplines needed are those of management services (operational research, systems analysis and cost/benefit planning), anthropology, epidemiology, biostatistics, economics, political science, environmental studies and law. All these tend to be poorly known in university clinical departments. All I can say is that efforts in these directions are slowly beginning. The real problem is that it is difficult to divert creative young scientists into such subjects merely because the 'Government' says that these subjects are those for which money will be made available. It is more important to recognize that it will take *time* to establish the necessary principles of creative research in these areas which cross so many disciplines.

Before we accept that people in university clinical departments 'need' to be diverted to different areas of research, I want to make one thing clear. We still practise medicine in an ocean of ignorance. At any fundamental level we know little about mental disease, arterial disease, emphysema, and even renal disease. Who should continue probing these areas if not people in university clinical departments?

I want now to mention our function as teachers. I am frankly horrified at the news that American medical schools are planning to turn out a high percentage of general practitioners. Our function surely is to produce a university graduate who has been imbued with the spirit of enquiry and critical analysis. Becoming a general practitioner (or anything else) is surely a matter for subsequent vocational training. If we fail to imbue our undergraduates with these qualities, then they will remain victims of the best advertiser for the remainder of their professional careers. The implications for health care and the drug bill are enormous!

The wave of feeling against academic research that has swept over our young people in the last few years has resulted in a reduction in the popularity of our departments. At the beginning of the 1960s, it was common for 20 or 30 people to apply for one lectureship; today, we are lucky if two or three apply. One can but hope that the 'backlash' to this anti-academic feeling will soon begin! Nevertheless, the increasing demands on us and the lack of popularity with young people have caused a sag in morale among the staff of these departments.

In conclusion, I suggest that we ought to look again at the idea of university hospitals. This idea was rejected in the UK, but such hospitals flourish in the USA and also in some Western European countries. They possess the great advantage of having a *whole* institution imbued with the ethos I have spoken about, rather than a small segment of an institution. It would be most important for such a university hospital to have a district function, for it would never flourish without a commitment to a defined community, nor would there ever be enough clinical material for undergraduate teaching. In our present economic situation, this idea must remain a dream, but I hope that during the next few years we shall see some critical evaluations of the efficacy (or otherwise) of the American university hospital, particularly in comparison with the British 'teaching' hospital.

Discussion

Roberts: Many successful preventive measures have been initiated without any detailed knowledge of related pathogenesis, for example, the dietary control of scurvy and the purification of faecally contaminated water to prevent cholera antedated by many years a proper understanding of the aetiological mechanisms of the diseases. We can expect with reasonable confidence that mortality from lung cancer and from ischaemic heart disease will be reduced once people change their smoking habits and diet and take exercise, well in advance of a proper understanding of the pathogenesis. Past experience has indicated that prevention relies on a substantial element of opportunism and empiricism—a point we should perhaps not lose sight of in our continuing search for the explanations of natural phenomena.

Guz: I entirely agree. Everything has grades of knowledge. There is no reason why we should not take preventive measures at all times. But the fact remains that until John Snow made the scientific observation about what happened at the water pump in London, ideas about cholera were nebulous. We talk about smoking and lung cancer now as if we have always known that they were related, but this was not so when I was a student—Hill and Doll had yet to do their brilliant biostatistical work to show it.

Roy: One can draw another conclusion from the quotations of Platt and Rosenheim: these two men are of acknowledged intelligence and perception and, therefore, there is a good chance that what they say about academics is relevant. Rosenheim also says[3] 'it must increasingly be the purpose of the medical profession and of all who work with them to aim at prevention rather than at cure'.

Birley: I agree; I believe that Platt's comments about some academics are correct. It is totally untrue to claim that all academic departments are full of people with burning curiosity—many are full of people who have run out of ideas. One may also say that many ordinary doctors spend a lot of time doing 'occupational therapy': the example may be cited of people looking at the recurrences of hernia. The criticism is not specific to academic departments. But one point that emerges from Dr Guz's paper is the nature of the other scientific variables that affect the course of illness. Much interest has centred on the physiological work on various organs and systems. Some people recognize a sigmoid growth curve in all subjects and perhaps traditional 'clinical science' has now passed the logarithmic phase. Hodgkin[4] demonstrated some years ago that the conditions which he saw as a student bore little relation to those he saw when he went into practice. Students now seem to have woken up to this fact and have become much more interested in what goes on outside hospitals. Many of these topics now need to be investigated scientifically by medical schools to complement what 'traditional academic' departments are doing.

Guz: I agree.

Tait: Dr Guz, you have described one reason why there seems to be a loss of interest in academic departments; one cannot have scientific medicine divorced from the social context of illness. As you said, the anthropological, ethical and political dimensions of research will have to be made scientific in relation to illness. The challenge to academic departments now is that they have to broaden their scientific base.

Guz: I agree.

Hockey: In this context, one cannot omit the Rothschild Report[5] in relation to research in the health service. With the emphasis on changing needs, it seems to me that now society not only gets the doctors it wants but it gets the research it wants. The Government is currently laying down priorities; in other words, it is telling us where we should concentrate our research but it is pre-empting the results of research by establishing priorities. I am anxious about this interference and the structure of the customer–contractor principle, although I can also see its potential for good.

Guz: I find myself again in agreement! The first signs of the winds of change came in the 1960s in Congress in the USA when people asked whether medical researchers were doing enough and whether money shouldn't be channelled into what people want. And how did the people express what they wanted?

Not through community health councils but presumably through their congressional leaders, so that the issue became political. Gradually this trend swept over the western world and Rothschild came out with a similar recommendation: the concept of the customer–contractor relationship, the idea that people at the top could define what was needed. Then came President Nixon's allocation of $500 000 000—a 'man-on-the-moon' programme—to wipe out cancer. But, on the whole, little has come from all this effort. Research depends on serendipity far too much, but that's the way it is. Why should anybody have wanted to know which way DNA was coiled? But somebody, supported by a benevolent Medical Research Council which was excited by the prospect, did just that and the whole of molecular biology emerged. Consequently, a lot of haematology has been clarified. I am glad that the Americans, who are rich compared to us, have tried the other way, especially as evidence from the USA indicates that their way may not be the way to do research. At the same time I can see no wrong in stating clearly what is not known and what are the prime needs. The issue of deciding where funds should go, which is the essence of the Congressional and Rothschild proposals, is a logical outcome, but will it lead to creative research?

Hockey: Do the community health councils know that they should or could influence research policy?

Guz: The Rothschild report came long before the reorganization of the National Health Service.

Knox: Dr Guz seems to have confused the kind of 'policy' initiated by Nixon with historical coalitions between medical scientists and special-interest consumer groups. In the USA and in most advanced countries including the UK, medical researchers have collaborated with consumers, with benefit to both, on special problems, such as those of paraplegics, parents of the mentally handicapped, cancer sufferers. Katz[6] traced the relationships between researchers, practitioners and consumers since the turn of the century. There now exists in the USA a medical science foundation almost entirely funded by community groups. Possibly community health councils will collectively evolve preferences and consequently influence the growth of particular areas of medical science, just as community controlled Health Maintenance Organizations in the USA have begun to link treatment priorities to resource allocations.[7]

Russell: Dr Guz, the medical education function was missing from your paper. Academic departments have another function, namely the development of new approaches and techniques for medical education. To do that, they have to take in all the points that Dr Tait and others have mentioned about what job they are trying to equip students for, and what skills they need to do it. Many academic departments seem not to have discussed this.

Guz: In undergraduate medical education I do not believe that what the consumer wants matters. That is the most antigenic remark I can make. At the postgraduate level, what the consumer wants and needs matters a great deal. I am making an extremely clear-cut distinction. We must produce some framework based on science in which to train medical graduates. Maybe we can shorten the curriculum from five to four years; of course, we should eliminate most of the dissection.

Paine: I was interested in your suggestion about university hospitals. It seems to me as an administrator that you were talking about units of excellence. Teaching hospitals have had the title of centres of excellence thrust upon them. Nevertheless, long ago the Goodenough report[8] seemed to suggest that the teaching hospital, with its tripartite function of providing a high standard of clinical service as well as teaching and research (duties which, especially in times of acute financial stringency, are often difficult to set in priority order), was too important to be put into an administrative system which was essentially service-orientated. That is why the teaching hospitals in England and Wales (undergraduate and postgraduate) were eventually given their own separate Boards of Governors when the National Health Service was implemented in 1948.

But we know that the undergraduate teaching hospitals also need districts because of the patients they provide, just as the districts need them for the services they give. Paradoxically, therefore, it seemed to me to be implicit in the recent reorganization of the National Health Service that the teaching hospitals are now considered too important to be left out of what is still essentially a service-oriented organization.

I tend, therefore, to conclude that perhaps teaching hospitals should be organized and administered in a completely different way which would recognize their academic status as well as their service function. Should all teaching hospitals in the UK become university hospitals? If so, is this a feasible proposition? Universities have never run hospitals here; they would have to form a link somehow with the health service.

Guz: And should they also remain district general hospitals? The idea has been tried in the USA.

Beckhard: Let me first clarify why the legislation pending in Congress that academic medical centres shall produce up to 50% generalists became a political power issue; it may relate to what is happening now in the UK. The issue, as I see it, in academic medicine is one of control of resources. Until about eight or nine years ago, the National Institutes of Health were the bank for the university medical centres providing research grants which supported many activities in medical schools. The dilemma of the mission of care of the medical centre— to produce new biomedical knowledge, to train doctors and to care for patients—

was resolved in favour of research. Then, the National Institutes of Health no longer had the resources to distribute. The public and the politicians had complained that too much money was being channelled into biomedical research.

This loss of funding made the heads of the university medical centres rethink their priorities. The issue became political rather than scientific or educational because of the maldistribution of doctors, the maldistribution of specialties, increased public pressure for more increased emphasis on primary care. It appeared that five years after their internship, graduates in internal medicine are in general practice and use their specialty less than 10% of their time. Similar facts have influenced greatly the debate about the training of an excess of specialists while many people do not have health care. The Federal goverment has stepped in by creating the National Health Service Corps. Legislation currently being considered will require a certain number of students to sign a contract when they start as medical students that they will serve two years after graduation in an underdeveloped area, working in general practice as part of a delivery team, otherwise the school will not receive government support for student tuition. So we have increased government 'interference' in the public sector. The politicians are taking on responsibilities that used to be shared between the consumers, the researchers and the academicians.

In academic medical centres the focus has now shifted from research to teaching as the primary objective. Every academic medical centre must now choose between being an academic medical *research* centre (producing graduates who will further the body of knowledge; the centre is, therefore, willing to lose certain kinds of government support and to face problems with the community) or an institution for teaching doctors—this means that primary care training is probably included in the first year curriculum of medical school and also that some basic research will be sacrificed.

Bridger: That is also happening in developing countries.

Roy: Yes; contrast East Africa with West Africa. In the West, separate university hospitals were developed usually on the periphery of large cities, leaving the government hospital to cope with the service needs of the urban population. The result has been disastrous for the health services. Elite students are being educated to become elite doctors while the ordinary citizen receives very poor service from an understaffed government hospital. In East Africa this did not happen; in both Nairobi and Kampala the teaching hospital was also the service hospital for the city and its surroundings. The concept of university hospitals must be qualified. Where they exist, they must also be the service hospital for the area.

A second point with developing countries is the question of how does one control doctors' training? For example, in Nairobi there were eight cardiologists and one cardiac surgeon. A government must step in to prevent such an imbalance. This is an interference in freedom, of course (and I am not clear myself about where the limits to this control should be set).

Baderman: Such state control has some attraction but it is the start of a dangerous road if one is not careful, because such decisions or influences may not always be based on purely numerical factors, but perhaps on political ones.

Bridger: In the argument about governmental control, for example, a step is being missed out for some reason—the failure of politicians to urge doctors to help put their own house in order.

Baderman: The politicians are at least as likely to get it wrong in that the basis of their decisions (such as, to limit the number of cardiologists) is often short-term expediency. They ought to ask, why are so many cardiologists wanting to get in on the act? Maybe the situation will be self-regulatory.

Guz: To reiterate; we must distinguish between undergraduate and postgraduate education. Dr Roy has been defining postgraduate education—a vocational training problem. I want a minimum norm, a core of knowledge, so that someone can learn to advance with what he has been taught. That to me is what a university hospital is all about, an undergraduate training centre.

Arie: All the topics that we believe are important—for instance, the issue of the individual patient as part of the total pool of potential users of the service—are as urgently in need of scientific study as are the subjects that Dr Guz is studying scientifically. One cannot divorce undergraduate from postgraduate education: as an undergraduate, the student is multipotential, most open to influence. His view of the purpose and nature of medical practice is set in innumerable unplanned ways, for instance by the implicit value systems of the university, by what the Professor of Medicine does *not* talk about, by the evident irritation of his teachers with certain unwanted patients or with old people 'blocking' beds. Education is as much a matter of attitudes as of imparting skills, of attitudes about what is worth doing, what is worth studying. The 'social' aspects of medicine are just as capable of being studied scientifically as the technical—though they are often more difficult and more elusive. Someone like Dr Guz could have a colossal influence both as an individual and *ex officio* as a Professor of Medicine if he could communicate these things, which I feel he is really in sympathy with. Instead of a polarity, there are vast areas of common ground.

Abercrombie: But Dr Guz is not presenting the common ground; what will come across to the student is the polarity.

Guz: I hope not, although it is a danger. The academic disciplines that I listed must be brought to bear on these crying problems. Where I must disagree (and I have Todd[9] and Merrison[10] on my side) is that there is a difference between undergraduate education and vocational training.

Birley: Merrison says that education is a continuous process. Regarding the subjects in the curriculum, I agree with you, but students are learning all sorts of things not in the curriculum, by imitation and by adopting the attitudes and unspoken beliefs of their teachers.

Baderman: I agree with Dr Guz a good deal, particularly about the strength of his feeling for the freedom and basic cohesive nature of undergraduate education, although it is obviously continuous and students are influenced by what happens in the postgraduate sector. He exemplified his point about the sanctity of the basic undergraduate education by the American experience of consciously directing at least a large part of undergraduate education from the start by financial constraints. If that is the basis of his anxiety, I am with him wholeheartedly.

Guz: I might add that my last three house physicians have left to take the steps towards going into general practice and, in spite of any 'evil influences' I may have exerted, I have done nothing but encourage them!

Roy: Academics seem to discuss medical education in totally unreal terms: in this country few if any of us have written down our objectives in any detail. In Nairobi, in response to a stimulus from WHO, I wrote down my objectives precisely, not just in vague terms such as 'we want a fully educated, highly intelligent doctor' but specifically 'that he should be able to read and interpret an electrocardiogram' and so on. From these, a curriculum could then be evolved. The Todd report[9] pretends to have set out objectives but they are still too vague and often mere clichés; I know of no department in a medical school in the UK that has made a realistic attempt to list its objectives. The head of a clinical academic department has a responsibility for the teaching of students throughout the clinical division. The students, however, receive disparate teaching from different clinicians who may not agree with the ideas of the Professor.

I am sure that you would agree, Dr Guz, that neither of us, however clear we may believe our objectives are, has any system of ensuring that our students learn what we think they should learn.

Guz: Yes. Multiple-choice questions do not give us the answer. The Merrison report tries harder than the Todd report to define objectives for the undergraduate, but the Todd report was the first attempt and so perhaps the use of clichés is more understandable.

Lucas: Isn't the problem of defining objectives important in the academic world in general?

Guz: Yes; but what about architecture? Like medicine, it has an academic phase followed by a vocational phase. Do the architectural schools in this country define their objectives?

Abercrombie: Some have tried. It seems that attempts to precede vocational training with the equivalent of a preclinical science do not have good effects on the students' learning to design.

Hockey: Objectives have been defined in nursing and maybe for once doctors could learn from us. In the post-basic Joint Board of Clinical Nursing Studies, for example, objectives are laid down for every single course: every procedure and type of preparation needed are described.

Arie: They also define their objectives in terms of attitudes as well as skills and knowledge. That is important.

Huntingford: On returning to an academic appointment earlier this year after four years with the WHO, I wrote a personal set of objectives, which I circulated to my colleagues. These were largely ignored by my hospital associates; I received no comments except from medical students and community physicians. One objective was to derive teaching objectives for my subject, obstetrics and gynaecology. I gained permission from the academic staff of the two medical colleges where I work to begin this exercise by drafting teaching objectives with the students. We have just completed this task. I now know why few, if any, medical schools have educational objectives. Our draft objectives were defined in terms of knowledge, skills and attitudes. The draft document provoked a hostile reaction from my colleagues, despite the fact that the objectives were drafted with their permission and were then submitted for their consideration. The students spent most of the time in drafting attitudinal objectives. This was a tremendously useful and interesting exercise. But it was the attitudinal objectives that were rejected in totality—including, for example, that one should not accept any clinical statement as a fact unless it was supported by evidence that students could weigh for themselves.

Guz: Who could fight that?

Huntingford: But it was rejected; that is why I am a revolutionary!

Baderman: The Joint Board experience, which I also shared (on the Accident and Emergency curriculum panel), was both illuminating, intimidating and foreign. (I am sure that my academic colleagues would not have found it as new as I did.) But as an exercise it occasionally seemed to be somewhat isolated from reality, perhaps because we were trying to design, in educational science terms, a curriculum for accident and emergency work. The difficulty will be in monitoring and assessing any educational programme which defines skills, knowledge and attitudes after it has been in operation.

Tait: Some years ago in Michigan State University medical educationalists tried hard to persuade the medical school to define specific educational objectives, but also tore the medical school apart trying to do this. What became apparent was that the nearer one approaches the heart of medicine the harder it is to define objectives in testable behavioural terms.

Roy: But my writing of objectives for my department in Kenya did work: I did not circulate it until I had shown it to all my surgical colleagues and had it accepted. Also, it was limited; it was not an exclusive list of objectives, but (as it must always be) open-ended and open to amendment. It formed the source from which the curriculum evolved and was accepted.[11] This was an easier task in Kenya than it is likely to be here because we decided that the purpose of undergraduate training was first to produce a district physician.

References

[1] FLEXNER, A. (1912) *Medical Education in Europe* (Report to the Carnegie Foundation), New York

[2] PLATT, R. (1967) Medical science: master or servant? *British Medical Journal 4*, 439–444

[3] ROSENHEIM, M. (1968) Health in the world of tomorrow. *Lancet 2*, 821–822

[4] HODGKIN, K. (1966) *Towards Earlier Diagnosis: A Family Doctor's Approach*, Livingstone, Edinburgh

[5] A Framework for Government Research and Development, presented to Parliament 1971 (1971) Cmnd. 4814 (Rothschild Report), HMSO, London

[6] KATZ, A.H. (1961) *Parents of the Handicapped*, pp. 136–150, E.C. Thomas, Springfield, Illinois

[7] SHEPS, C.G. (1972) The influence of consumer sponsorship on medical services. *Milbank Memorial Fund Quarterly L*, 4 (II)

[8] MINISTRY OF HEALTH AND DEPARTMENT OF HEALTH FOR SCOTLAND (1944) *Interdepartmental Committee on Medical Schools (Goodenough Committee): Report*, HMSO, London

[9] ROYAL COMMISSION ON MEDICAL EDUCATION, 1965–1968 (1968) *Report* (Cmnd. 3569), HMSO, London

[10] REPORT OF THE COMMITTEE OF INQUIRY INTO THE REGULATION OF THE MEDICAL PROFESSION (1975) (Cmnd. 6081) HMSO, London

[11] ROY, A.D. (1969) Surgical training in East Africa. *East African Medical Journal 6*, 1–8

Health education, cancer and postgraduate training

GRAHAM JOYSON

The Royal Marsden Hospital, London

Abstract Cancer as a term encompasses a multitude of diseases and is consequently misunderstood. Today, it is still considered sinister and, too often, synonymous with death. It is a complex subject, exciting and challenging, yet the myths associated with cancer are perpetuated even by professionals in the health service. This can be attributed to the scant knowledge of its nature and prognosis, the progress made and the services available. When one considers the breadth of basic training needed to prepare both doctors and nurses to practise it is understandable.

In a health service based on disease it is difficult to consider prevention as a priority. Financial implications are enormous and inhibit this aspect of the work in the field of cancer and allied diseases. However, it is estimated that 80–90% of cancers are caused by environmental influences and can, in theory, be prevented. Efforts to promote health and prevent disease are costly and too often ineffective.

Early diagnosis is another contentious subject; efforts are being directed to the establishment of clinics for patients presenting with symptoms rather than detection of symptom-free subjects. Improved approaches to prevention, recognition and acceptance through an understanding of cancer will alleviate the task of those directly involved in the cure and control of the disease.

Health education in relation to cancer needs to be directed equally at health service professionals and the public.

It would be unacceptable and inaccurate to describe the cancer services anywhere as incapable of further improvement. Research and therapy must go hand in hand and depend on the participation of the patient as a knowledgeable member of the team, rather than as a passive recipient of care. Death should not be considered failure, rather the completion of care.

We face constantly the risk of despondency and the efforts of the team must be sustained with optimism and encouragement. Achievements have been made and will be made, however slowly, and the end justifies the effort. The need for postgraduate training is greater now than ever before. Adaptability to rapid change, vision and continuity are vital in our technologically orientated society. This should be considered a prerequisite to ensure improved standards of patient care at home and in hospital.

143

HEALTH EDUCATION

When in 1851 Dr William Marsden founded the Free Cancer Hospital—the first hospital in the world to be devoted exclusively to the treatment of cancer—the prosperity and affluence of Victorian England were at their height. So, too, were the ignorance and prejudice of the average citizen towards poverty and disease. It was these enemies—and the constant lack of funds—which dogged the efforts of the dedicated Dr Marsden from the outset. Nevertheless, when he died in 1867, his enthusiasm and passionate ideals had begun to make inroads into the opinions and purses of influential society.

At the first meeting of the Governors in 1851 Dr Marsden said 'Now Gentlemen, I want to found a hospital for the treatment of cancer and for the study of the disease, for at the present time we know absolutely nothing about it'. Thus from the very first the Hospital has been concerned not only with the treatment but with research and teaching.

The intervening 124 years have seen much progress made and today we know a great deal more about the diseases. Unfortunately, they are insidiously innocent in onset and remain difficult to diagnose. Many of them have become easy to manage but some are still bewildering and complex in both presentation and aetiology. It is distressing to note that the general concept of cancer bears little resemblance to its reality. Far too many people are unfamiliar with its true cause, nature, prognosis and the treatment available and this is reflected amongst professionals in the health service themselves. As the second most significant killer disease in the country it deserves interest and commands our attention. My thesis is that we urgently need to educate the 'professionals' in parallel with the public.

As nurses we have a unique contribution to make in assisting the patient, both in sickness and in health. There is now, throughout the world, among all sorts and conditions of men, the knowledge that poverty and disease are not inevitable.

The World Health Organization in 1946 gave the following definition: 'Health is a state of complete physical, mental and social well being, and not merely the absence of disease and infirmity'. How many of us today can claim to meet these criteria in an ever more stressful society? The difficulty is increased when we see the population so seldom anxious to pursue healthy precepts if it means refraining from unhealthy but pleasurable stimuli.

Research and trials have produced absolute methods of control in some diseases, the re-emergence of which illustrates the negative attitude to the observation of even the simplest available precautions. This applies in particular to communicable diseases.

Occupational hazards, to some extent, are obviated by the onus of responsibility being placed on employers to ensure safe working conditions for their employees. Radiation hazards in industry and hospital are known and elaborate precautions are taken to prevent accidents. The disadvantage is that owing to the unseen nature of radiation, warnings and measures of protection are too frequently ignored.

The mass media have supported campaigns which highlight risks, but there is little evidence of improved health as a direct result. To a certain extent we tend to expect too much of an already overloaded community service. So far, we have been unable to match need and demand in the community by our avid concentration on the acutely sick in the adventure-packed setting of a hospital. The more dependent the population becomes, the less concerned it will be to face its responsibility for its own health.

Whilst propagating health education in relation to cancer, I am conscious of the alarmist effect of too much information. For instance, many screening clinics became quickly oversubscribed owing to the success of the educational effort and publicity. This in turn can create psychological trauma and thus a new but real problem. There are many dangers in offering a service in isolation, especially in times of financial stringency. Any health programme should be fully financed and continue to ensure optimum usage and effect. It is useless to inject funds on a one-off basis without any assurance of continuity and progress. My question is, therefore, whether we should disclose new findings or facilities before we are confident of their availability to all. The time for the isolated health project is over; a global view needs to be taken. Whatever is planned, any future delivery of health care systems should be a part of the overall health programme of the country.

Much needs to be done to educate the public to a better understanding of health. The setting up of Regional Cancer Councils should help to pinpoint deficiencies as far as practicable. These councils recognize that in many areas clinicians are overworked, there are gaps in communication and financial limits on expenditure and the councils hope to assist in detecting and remedying inadequacies within these limitations. Patients' attitudes to cancer are determined by the attitude to the disease by the public in general.

Far too often by the time cancer is diagnosed, the disease has already been present for many months or years.

How can this situation be prevented? Our objectives are threefold: to discover when and from what cause a tumour originates; to identify the factors that hasten or retard its early growth; and to perfect methods of early detection.

In cancer of the lung and the bladder, the causes of which are largely known, there is still much to be done, even if the main action needed now is social or legislative persuasion.

The remaining forms of human cancer—that is the vast majority of cancers, including those affecting the breast, stomach, colon and blood—present a bewildering variety of problems, both in causes and detection. Although progress in this field has been disappointingly slow, new methods are emerging by which it is hoped that positive conclusions will eventually be reached.

Xeroradiography, mammography and thermography are well established and may show up otherwise undetectable tumours of the breast. The use of computer facilities to feed in data on indicants of risk will help to streamline this service and identify the most appropriate diagnostic tool for individuals. Cytology may perhaps enable us to identify individuals at particular risk— especially if methods can be improved for the study of enzymes, chromosomes and other cell characteristics in greater detail.

In some cases hormone assays may indicate the person prone to cancer and, should it be proved that viruses play a role in human cancer, immunological or other means may be successful in identifying the virus-infected cell which may be the starting point of a tumour. Meanwhile, the search for quicker and more sensitive methods of detection goes on.

CANCER

I can only give a brief account of the progress being made and of the magnitude of the problems that remain. This disease, for example, is still responsible for one quarter of all deaths of people between the ages of 15 and 44. But methods of treatment are continually being improved and, through new skills and more advanced techniques, it is possible to diagnose and cure cancer, especially in the early stages, in more and more patients. It is only by painstaking research and the efforts of dedicated people in this country and elsewhere that the scourge of cancer will be finally defeated.

In the health services today we have not reached the happy state of fully involving our patients although more clinicians are making an effort to work with rather than simply on behalf of the patient. The nursing profession feels it is not a question of what patients should be told but one of how to tell them. Concentration on individual assessment is vital but it is evident that most patients want to have what they suspect or know to be true confirmed. Unfortunately, it is not simple: one can hardly tell the patient that he has cancer and then make no further reference to his treatment and prognosis. For many, the truth is easy since the outlook is good; for others, the prognosis is poor but it is nonetheless important to discuss—the effects of treatment in cancer are often far worse than the symptoms with which the patients present. In the USA it is a legal requirement to give full information to the patient, but one must remember that there the public are much more litigation conscious and the clinicians litigation nervous. Nonetheless, support for cancer research is outstanding. The American National Cancer Research Fund has risen from $180 000 000 in 1970 to $699 000 000 in 1975. Perhaps this is an indication of the benefit of better health education and the arousal of the public's interest. In this country the patients' 'ostrich'-like quality of burying their heads in the sand can partly be attributed to mimicry of the even worse 'ostrich' syndrome adopted by the professions.

Patients themselves can often make a most useful and significant contribution to their treatment. I am convinced that shrouding the treatment in mystique is a disservice to ourselves and open to misinterpretation or loss of confidence in us by the patients. At the Royal Marsden, we constantly advocate participation but this cannot be effective without the patient as a member of the team. This is not a problem exclusive to oncology, but cancer exacerbates the situation because of its connotations, real or apparent. Nursing staff in general tend to encourage dependence rather than independence of the patient. Unfortunately, there is still the attitude among some hospital nursing staff that the ward is their enclave and, as such, sacrosanct. However, it has been said that today nurses can analyse and synthesize but can no longer catheterize! We aim to standardize team concepts of nursing or case assignment to facilitate total patient care and increase the nurses' satisfaction.

The incidence of cancer in this country is increasing. This is partly attributable to longevity since successful antibiotic regimes have reduced the risks associated with hitherto 'killer diseases' of the aged. Longevity has produced and is still producing new problems, of which cancer is only one. The health services are faced with an ever increasing 'disposal' problem, which refers rather rudely to patients occupying beds without needing to be kept in hospital. Although many of these patients could easily be cared for in the family, they are seen as a nuisance and as disrupting a changed life style. Patients' feelings of guilt connected with disease exacerbate the problem for those dealing with cancer; elderly patients, in particular, think of themselves as dirty or anti-social. The number of patients who present with such advanced disease that the only possible approach is palliation is a sad reflection on the 'system' and difficult to accept as inevitable.

POST-BASIC TRAINING

As the need for post-basic training has been recognized it is no longer looked upon as a luxury for the privileged few; instead, it should be considered as an essential part of professional development if we are to maintain and improve our standards of care.

To meet these increasing demands of post-basic education for nurses and to standardize training nationally, the Joint Board of Clinical Nursing Studies was established in 1969. It was decided that a course in cancer nursing was needed and in 1973 a specialist panel was set up to produce an outline curriculum, approved in 1974. The courses are based to a large extent on courses previously arranged by individual specialist hospitals to meet their own needs. Today, we have the advantage of a nationally agreed curriculum and a method of certification of successful course members acceptable to all hospitals which gives the standardization so necessary in these days of high mobility of labour.

The course is designed to cover all aspects of oncology and we hope to train a nurse who, on completion of the course, is knowledgeable and skilled in all aspects of care relating to malignant disease. She will recognize the value and contribution that the various types of treatment make to the cure of cancer and understand that, when cancer is not curable, valuable palliation may be achieved.

The material covered by the course includes the nature of cancer, carcino-genesis and the environmental factors relating to malignant disease, methods of detection, the principles of treatment, and the specific needs of the different age groups, including children.

During the course we expect our students to begin to identify patients' problems and assess their needs so that they will be able to provide resources and facilities to meet individual physical, social and spiritual needs of the patient. One aim is to return the patient to society as independent as possible and, therefore, an understanding of the principles of rehabilitation and of the part the nurse can play to support other members of the caring professions, such as physiotherapists and social workers, is essential in helping the patient to cope with any defects that he may have as a result of his disease or treatment.

We have observed that our nurses quickly become sensitive to cues given by patients and their families with regard to their individual needs and fears. It seems safe to assume that the more conversant the patient is about his role the more he will facilitate the roles of the various people engaged in his therapy.

Cancer centres have had an advantage and a disadvantage over general hospitals. For a long time, many nurses have thought of cancer hospitals as terminal-care homes or, at best, homes for the incurable. Attitudes towards the care of cancer patients have changed and a much more optimistic view is now expressed. We have been able to gain some advantage from past pessimism in the care of our terminal patients. The nursing-care plans and policies for this group of patients in our cancer hospitals are probably more advanced than in any other sphere of medicine. Not that our patients need better care —observation of patients dying from neuromuscular disorders or chronic bronchitis reminds us that their needs are often far greater than those of the cancer patient—but we have been able to set standards for this type of care that can be modelled by other specialties. We stress the importance of helping the patient to develop and maintain the maximum capacity for normal living to obtain the fullest quality of life. We also stress the importance of preserving the dignity of the patient and the acceptance of the inevitability of death. Death should be looked upon not as a failure of our care but rather as the completion of our care.

In management our main concern is with training for the management of patient care; how to form nursing assessments of patients; to make individual goals and objectives for patients that are measurable and attainable; how to plan a patient's day and his clinical care during that period, and the overall nursing plan leading to his transfer home to his family or into the care of the community services.

Teaching the patient to care for himself is the most effective nursing procedure, and teaching relatives is of equal importance.

If the professional standards of nursing are to be maintained, an understanding of the principles of basic research and clinical research methods is desirable. Nursing today cannot be based solely on past traditions. We must be able to evaluate our practice and procedures and to develop new procedures and techniques. If we are to improve our present standards of nursing care, we must constantly review our present care systems; an appreciation of research methods is valuable in making an objective assessment of alternative nursing-care programmes.

In summary, with regard to the aims and objectives of post-basic training in oncological nursing, we hope to attain a standard of care for our patients that is in keeping with rapid developments and improvements in medical technology.

Naturally, we do not restrict our training to these lengthy, specialized courses. Present opinion seems to favour shorter courses but the prerequisite is that they should be recognized. We do not expect all nurses caring for cancer patients to attend the course, for most cancer patients are cared for in general hospitals or the community and in these circumstances constitute only a part of the wide range of responsibilities. To meet the needs of this group we have to arrange several programmes. Our community colleagues are catered for by a series of two-day workshops arranged in conjunction with the Queen's Institute of District Nursing, Chiswick Polytechnic and the hospital. Although, at present, the workshops are attended by experienced district nurses, those in training and hospital nurses, we hope to convert them into interdisciplinary sessions for all members of the primary health care team. We have arranged to hold one-week refresher courses for health visitors. This is another joint venture between the Royal Marsden Hospital and the Council for the Education and Training of the Health Visitor, and these courses commenced in September, 1975.

I ought to mention the programme that we have to ensure we keep our own house in order. It is too simple for our own senior staff to slip into complacency by losing touch with developments in other specialist areas. We tend to concentrate on clinical subjects but with these we couple study days on management topics to ensure a well balanced professional development. The mid-day study sessions organized by the medical clinical tutor are attended by as many nursing as medical staff. These are particularly useful in fostering the right relationships between the professions.

Naturally, we have a long way to go to achieve all our goals but we feel we are approaching the problems from the right direction. Many specialist centres and hospitals are undertaking similar programmes and we should welcome constructive suggestions to help us to continue our work in a meaningful way. We seem to be a long way from the establishment of group sessions with our patients. This surely could be overcome with a positive approach to the problem of telling and, in telling, supporting and following through.

The health of a family, a group or a people depends on the sharing of feelings of anxiety and guilt, as well as joy and acceptance.[1]

Discussion

Lucas: How much scope is there in their educational activities for the nursing staff to ventilate their anxieties and feelings? This seems to be a borderline area between psychotherapy and education.

Joyson: There is full scope and we encourage this. The greatest conflict among nurses is always attributed to problems of communication. For instance, nurses now believe that the patient should be told but we are wondering how to tell them (p. 146). The medical profession have traditionally accepted the role of the teller and the nursing staff are not anxious to take this over unless they are given *carte blanche* to do so. The conflict arises from not knowing what the patient has been told, even though we now have a system in which a consultant can record what is said to the patient.

Birley: Another aspect of our guilt is our enthusiasm for doing something regardless of its efficacy—for instance, are we being ostrich-like about the facts on preventive work? What is the evidence that screening the breast and cervix is of any use?

Joyson: Many facilities are already in existence but in the present economic climate there is little support for the screening of symptom-free subjects as such; there is much more interest in setting up symptom-based clinics as early diagnostic units.

Certainly there is controversy about how effective screening procedures are. We identify six suspicious cases per 1000 by screening the breast and cervix but when a patient presents with a malignant lump in a breast it is estimated that it has been developing for at least 10 years. Every patient who comes with a lump is biopsied; biopsy is the only sure way of diagnosis in this type of disease. We have now restricted screening to women of age 35 or older and this has caused psychological torment to younger women. It is alleged that in Japan screening has dramatically reduced the number of deaths due to cancer of the stomach; doctors can now cope with the disease in its early stages. I would press for screening in the future not only for the breast.

Huntingford: A traditional role that the medical (and nursing) profession has given itself is reassurance. I am concerned about telling people something that it is not the truth as we perceive it but what we think is necessary for reassurance. This is particularly difficult when there can be no reassurance.

Joyson: We try to tell them the truth (not only to reassure them) and bring them into the team with the medical staff, the paramedical staff and the nurses, so that it is a supportive group. In the USA, patients take part in group sessions; since they know about their illnesses they meet and talk out their problems together.

Huntingford: Do you tell the patient in a group?

Joyson: No, we tell them individually first and then set up groups.

Huntingford: Can you be sure of the attitudes of those who tell them? Can you be sure that false reassurance is not given?

Joyson: At the moment, no, although the nursing staff are geared to this. Medical staff in the chemotherapy section where much research goes hand in hand with treatment are particularly skilled at this, but by then, patients know about their condition and their treatment. In other areas, consultants find it difficult to cope with this problem, especially in the terminal care unit where they appear, to the patient, to be rejecting them. Patients admitted to the terminal care unit may come under the aegis of a pain consultant who manages their pain adequately; the nursing staff look after all the basic needs, but the consultant who has been in charge of them for many years might never even drop in to see them. We do not want to look on death as a failure, we want to look on it as the completion of care.

Abercrombie: You seemed to imply that the consultant's message was given once and understood immediately. I noticed how patients in the cerebral palsy paediatric unit at Guy's Hospital would ask the nurses to explain what the doctor had clearly said. There seem to be two aspects of communication: stating the truth, with or without overtones about reassurance, and digesting and comprehending this information, which may take months. This is done better in collaboration with peers amongst whom there may be more free discussion and less authoritarian statements about what one should believe. The respective roles of the nurse and consultant are not opposite but complementary.

Joyson: That is just what we are trying to achieve.

Bickerton: Nurses are now being trained to discuss frankly with patients and relatives, so that the relative can help the patient—it is a combined effort. But nurses often do not know how much the patient has been told or how he was told. The same terminology prevails throughout a hospital but when the nurse is asked, say, in the home whether a person has cancer, she is in difficulty. Has the general practitioner also been asked? If so, what did he say? What should the nurse say? We must agree on a procedure for such patients. We inform patients when they have had a myocardial infarction and can discuss the treatment. Can we not do the same with the cancer patient? In a survey by the Tavistock Institute,[2] patients were asked whether they knew what they were suffering from; 90%, although it had never been discussed, knew that they had cancer but were never in a position to discuss it with their next of kin.

Joyson: In the paediatric oncology unit, we have now a team consisting of a health visitor, a district nursing sister based in the hospital working together with the hospital medical and nursing staff, the general practitioner and the medical social worker. Problems in paediatric oncology, particularly with siblings, are being alleviated by the health visitor and community nursing sister —there is continuity of care and much better communication. In general, one cannot tell a patient once and expect him to remember for all time without supporting him and following it through.

Tait: We ought to remember that denial often operates to protect patients; doctors may decide what to say but the patient decides what he will take in. It can be most distressing to summon up courage to tell the truth to a patient only to find oneself back where one started. Dying can be such a painful problem that there is often no way in which we, too, can escape the pain. Our task is then to show that we can bear it.

Arie: We tend to imply that if only medical staff would tackle the problem in the right way, all would be well. There we are on treacherous ground. Studies of uptake of information by patients have shown how complex it is. Hinton[3] found that many dying patients were aware and had accepted that they were dying without this having been explicitly discussed. Aitken-Swan & Easson[4] carefully told patients with 'curable' cancers (e.g. skin cancers) the nature of their disease but, a few weeks later, found that nearly 20% of them denied having been told. Hugh-Jones et al.[5] made a special attempt to give patients systematic information about the hospital, their treatment and their diagnosis and its implications. When the patients were subsequently interviewed, a month after discharge, 40% were dissatisfied with the information they had been given. Ley & Spelman[6] studied processes of giving and receiving information in more detail. Joyce[7] published a paper about communication with patients with the eloquent title: 'What does the doctor let the patient tell him?' So much of communication consists of covert messages about what one is willing to hear. There *are* instances when it is wrong to give information to patients. There are even exceptional circumstances in which doctors should resist demands for further opinions.

Roy: Doctors, particularly the least secure doctors, do resist requests for second opinions. So, as a general principle, a second opinion requested by a patient should always be encouraged and courteously granted. I do, however, understand what you mean.

Arie: I am sure that we all agree that we should make it extremely easy for patients to get second opinions but I am thinking of, say, the family with a dying child who go for the fifth or sixth opinion. Sometimes, it is the doctor's duty to take on himself, so to speak, the guilt for saying no, thereby perhaps preventing the family ruining itself financially and emotionally in pursuing hopeless cures. When the child dies, the family can feel that they were willing to leave no stone unturned but were stopped by the doctor, rather than accusing themselves of not having done enough. These instances are exceptional, but they do exist. Similarly, there are exceptional occasions when one should systematically attempt not to give the patient information. Patients sometimes give clues, either directly or in other ways, or by what they do not say, that they don't want to know. I have been involved in a few 'successful' deaths (and I agree with Mr Joyson that death can be the successful conclusion of care), when the patient never knew he or she was dying, and I was sure that it was right that way.

Roy: But the signal to you to say that they did not want to know meant that they did know. Surely, what happens most often is that when the doctor has contact with the patient over a long time, the patient knows that he has cancer, the doctor knows that he knows, but the patient does not want it put into words. The patient may have the same relationship with his relatives. This has the advantage that, in moments of despair, the patient can imagine that he was wrong because it has never been explicitly stated; one leaves him with the capacity to assuage despair by hope.

Arie: I accept that entirely. Often one sees an extraordinary and almost biological force in doctors who are dying—a denial, which is not necessarily maladaptive, with which one has to acquiesce despite one's instinct to give information. We must comply with those doctors who, by any rational criterion, must know what is happening but are somehow able not to know.

Baderman: We are in danger of expunging or attempting to expunge our guilt for past misdemeanours of not telling patients by feeling that we must tell everybody everything all the time. I agree with Dr Arie. Part of the overall assessment of patients is not only what is the matter with them but what they think is the matter with them and what they want us to tell them at a particular time. Telling is not a once-and-for-all transaction. Also, one must be careful what one tells a patient who, for instance, comes into an accident department with a crushing chest pain and the old fashioned *angor animi*, the fear of impending dissolution, even though one may be certain that he has had a massive myocardial infarction and may be going to die soon. One needs not only an electrocardiogram but as much information as possible from him and his relatives to decide what to say, what to say to the nurses and how much to say the next day. Colleagues have been known to rush in and say 'well, you have had a heart attack, old man, but you will be all right'—the last part comes too late because after the first part of the sentence the patient goes into ventricular fibrillation and dies.

The decision to tell entails more than just description of the diagnosis; as doctors, we have now come to accept that we have a responsibility. The patient may ask about the implications of the diagnosis, treatment and the likely outcome. With regard to outcome, sometimes we do not know which treatment to use let alone whether it will be successful. Outcome may be uncertain. The complexity of 'telling' should inhibit us from adopting blanket policies or radical attitudes, however theoretically proper.

Levitt: Whose health is it that we are talking about? Whose illness is it? I don't minimize the responsibilities that doctors, nurses and others face in treating patients but their assumption that they possess the patient's illness and that it is for them to deal with it as they think best may not be right, particularly in view of Dr Arie's comments about second opinions and withholding information. The patient may be badly equipped to handle his illness but that is his responsibility and it is the doctor's responsibility to teach him how to do that.

Paine: As the aphorism says, no-one dies of a disease, they die of their whole life. Michael Wilson suggests[8] that the prime function of a hospital is to teach people that the miracles of medical science are somewhat limited and that illness is very much a part of living. Mr Joyson, do you at times bring chaplains into the therapeutic team?

Joyson: To a certain extent we do, for in our hospital the chaplain set up an interdisciplinary group, which is one of the most effective groups for getting action within the hospital on patient-care policies; it includes medical staff, nursing staff, paramedical staff and is run by the chaplain. The chaplain has been most useful because of his approach to care.

Bickerton: Relatives have an awful burden to carry. It has been and still is practice for relatives to be told and for that reason the group discussion with the relatives at St. Christopher's Hospice in South London shows that one can train people to accept the inevitable. Consequently, they can face the facts. Nurses now, with their extra training, can perhaps look at death, for instance, in a different light.

Joyson: We base what we say to the patient on individual assessment. Part of our training enables us to become sensitive to cues from patients we know well; we know whom we can tell. Only a few cannot be told.

Hockey: I agree with Miss Levitt. A patient has the right to ask the person from whom he can accept the information and that may not always be the doctor, but a nurse, an auxiliary or another member of the team in whom the patient has confidence. We found this repeatedly in our study *Life Before Death.*[9]

Do doctors realize what harm they do themselves in playing confidence tricks? For example, consider a doctor who tells a member of the family but not the patient that the patient has cancer. I interviewed hundreds of such people. In one instance the daughter complained that she could not now believe her doctor if he told her that the lump in her breast was benign, as he had told her that her mother had cancer while encouraging the mother by saying it was all right. Often the doctors neither realize nor acknowledge that kind of effect of such a policy.

Roy: We seem to be enunciating a principle that we shall only tell the patient the truth; we must decide, therefore, whether the patient wants or needs the truth at any particular time. In the past, we have talked to patients but not told them the truth.

Bridger: This topic is central to everybody and we are all as much involved on the receiving end as the people we are talking about but we seem to be using this session as a window through which we can look at UK health needs in a changing setting. The themes that then stand out most are the role of the patient in the total care team—the different ways and methods of teaching, and the relationship of the patient and the hospital to the community. Although these themes have been concerned principally with cancer and the work that is being done at the Royal Marsden Hospital, we should recognize their wider and general significance.

References

[1] WILSON, M. (1975) *Health is for People*, Darton, Longman & Todd, London
[2] BALINT, M. *et al.* (1970) *Treatmen. or Diagnosis: Study of Repeat Prescriptions in General Practice*, Tavistock Publications, London
[3] HINTON, J. (1963) The physical and mental distress of the dying. *Quarterly Journal of Medicine 32*, 1
[4] AITKEN-SWAN, J. & EASSON, E. C. (1959) Reactions of cancer patients on being told their diagnosis. *British Medical Journal 1,* 783
[5] HUGH-JONES, P., TANSER, A. R. & WHITBY, C. (1964) Patient's view of admission to a teaching hospital. *British Medical Journal 2*, 660–664
[6] LEY, P. & SPELMAN, M.S. (1967) *Communicating with the Patient*, Staples Press, London
[7] JOYCE, C.R.B. (1964) What does the doctor let the patient tell him? *Journal of Psychosomatic Research 8*, 343–352
[8] WILSON, M. (1971) *Hospital, a Place of Truth: Study of the Role of the Hospital Chaplain*, University of Birmingham Institute for the Study of Relative Architecture, Birmingham
[9] CARTWRIGHT, A., HOCKEY, L. & ANDERSON, J.L. (1973) *Life Before Death*, Routledge and Kegan Paul, London

Women and their health: is there a conflict?

PETER HUNTINGFORD

Joint Academic Unit of Obstetrics, Gynaecology and Reproductive Physiology, The London Hospital Medical College and The Medical College of St. Bartholomew's Hospital, London

Abstract Women play a dual role in society that demands special consideration not only of women themselves but also for the sake of their children, their male partners (if any), families as a whole, and society in general. From a consideration of the health needs of women and how they affect their status in society, the following objectives are considered essential for the development of health services in support of the rights of women and human rights in general: the importance of the dual role of women in society and their struggle for freedom to choose whether they exercise a reproductive function must be recognized; individuals must be provided with the means to control their own fertility; individual women must be given the information and means necessary to protect their own health; and health services must play their part in gaining equality of status, opportunity and contribution of women to society. The conflicts arise from the way in which women are treated: they are not treated as equals either as colleagues or as people seeking health services; they are denied the right to control their own fertility; they are not consulted sufficiently as consumers of the services offered. The major primary constraint to the resolution of these conflicts is the attitude of those responsible for providing health services to women. Only secondarily do women increase the constraint by acquiescence to the attitudes of those serving them.

A DOCTOR'S ATTITUDE TO CHANGE

My own attitudes have been shaped by my experience as an obstetrician and gynaecologist faced with personal conflicts arising from my interests in fetal medicine, abortion, teaching medical students and an interlude of four years in Asia with the World Health Organization as an associate of nationals at central government level concerned with the planning of birth control programmes.

In many ways I have been disillusioned by my experiences. In Dr Abercrombie's terms I have recognized my egocentricity and the need—my need—to accept the fact that 'observer error' exists. I felt that Dr Abercrombie[1] was providing me with an excuse to stop asking questions, that she was saying 'realize that there is a degree of change which eventually nobody can accept' and 'to tolerate change, it is legitimate to deceive yourself'. Whether she meant that is of little importance since the result has been to strengthen my resolve not to deceive myself, to continue asking questions, and to press for my own limit of tolerance of change. I have found life easier since I have deliberately sought change and denied boundaries.

I have been forced to question my own attitudes, because I was fortunate to be working with a group of consumers who have raised and continue to raise their voices in questioning the attitudes of myself and others like me who wish to care for them. Sooner or later, we realize that this wish cannot be fulfilled by care alone, but only if we also know what is wanted by those for whom we care. Throughout this symposium the consumers have appeared but I would submit that they have done so only as one of the images observed by Escher in his silver ball (cf. p. 12). Consumers have not appeared at the focal point of our discussions. Until we are able to perceive the needs of consumers from their egocentric point of view, we shall never satisfy them.

Discussion of cost–benefit analyses and similar indices without any account being taken of consumer satisfaction cannot measure completely the achievement of the health services.

CONFLICT BETWEEN WOMEN AND THE HEALTH SERVICES

Much of the present conflict within the National Health Service that we are currently facing in the UK derives from our failure as professionals to expand our egocentric view and an insistence that our view is the correct one.

The conflicts existing between women and those caring for their health illustrate the gap between the thinking of the professionals and that of consumers. In the medical professions it is generally assumed that all women want to be mothers, that infertility and childlessness bring unhappiness, that those women who do not share these attitudes either totally or in part are not quite normal, that women who find themselves pregnant and reject the situation are irresponsible not to have foreseen and avoided the possibility, and that safety and health have the same meaning for everyone.

Why do we make such sweeping generalizations and assumptions? Why do we reject, and often not even listen to, suggestions from those whom our assumptions concern? Perhaps it is because we need the comfortable confines of recognizable boundaries and even the safety of barriers when we feel really threatened.

THE ROLE OF WOMEN IN SOCIETY

In theory, women can exercise one of two, or both, roles in society: a reproductive role, as the mother of children, and as an individual contributor without regard to gender. Until now most women have not been able to choose: they have been mothers (or were left on the shelf), whilst inequality of opportunity and status prevented the full development and use of their contributions as individuals to society. At last, an increasing number of women in this country are able to choose for themselves from the options of acting an exclusive role as mothers, a dual role as mothers and as individuals, or of declining their reproductive function and pursuing equally with men a role in society that is independent of their sex.

Real choice between these options, however, cannot exist until such time as the means for all women to choose are made available. Such means include: equal opportunities for education and employment; ready access to contraceptives and abortion; protection of employment during childbearing and motherhood; recognition that motherhood is an experience of life equivalent to uninterrupted employment; facilities for the day-care of children; support for one-parent families, etc.

THE HEALTH NEEDS OF WOMEN

Women have some special health needs distinct from those of men. This must be recognized if the health services are to provide support for the achievement of women's rights. Women need care during pregnancy, childbirth and while their children are dependent; they need specialized technical services to deal with diseases peculiar to women and the means to prevent conception and cope with unwanted pregnancies. In the provision of these services, women's needs must be perceived and understood, and women must be treated as equals with respect, dignity and sensitivity.

THE TYPES OF CONFLICT

The number, variety and often paradoxical nature of conflicts that exist between women and those providing obstetric and gynaecological services are evidence that the needs of women are neither being listened to nor understood. Examples of these conflicts are well known to formal groups of consumers such as the Consumers' Association, the Patients' Association for the Improvement of Maternity Services and the National Childbirth Trust, as well as to individual women and to informal groups. The conflicts relate to the provisions for contraception and abortion, to the prolonged investigation of infertility, to the investigation and treatment of vaginal discharge and recurrent urinary tract infections, to difficulties with sexual intercourse and menopausal symptoms, to attitudes towards operations such as sterilization and hysterectomy, to the desire by some women to return to home confinement, to the induction and acceleration of labour, to the increasing use of scientific equipment, potent analgesics and anaesthetics, and of obstetric intervention during delivery, to the arbitrary use of routines of unproven value such as prolonged stay in hospital, pubic shaves, enemata, the separation of mothers and babies for observation, delay in the establishment of infant suckling, and to confusion of advice given especially about breast-feeding and contraception.

THE CAUSES OF CONFLICT

In all these conflicts between women and the profession, I feel that the underlying cause is a defensive reaction on the part of doctors to fears that their image, role and status in society are threatened. To prevent change doctors claim that they know best; their expertise, skills and opinions cannot be properly examined and questioned from outside without so-called clinical independence and freedom being destroyed and interference with the relationship between doctor and patient. No data are provided to support these claims. Objective evaluation by outside observers of medical activities is prohibited. Criticisms and even questions often provoke irrational responses. Doctors, by imposing their own professional values through the advice that they give, prevent other people from contributing to and broadening the base of the teaching and learning opportunities offered during medical consultations. Doctors generally find it easier to talk than to listen—hence, my mistrust of counselling. The medical profession demonstrates a reluctance to accept new roles as exemplified by the hairsplitting arguments about whether the provision of family planning services is a medical or social activity. Surely the whole of medical care is a social activity. Generally, doctors underestimate the ability of lay people to understand and to participate in medical decisions, which justifies the denial to lay people of full information and of the ability to take responsibility for themselves. The use of elaborate jargon is essential to perpetuate the argument that the public are ignorant and incapable, and to justify continuing defensive attitudes. Beyond this, doctors suffer new anxieties about whether to use techniques recently made available. Anxiety about the use of the technique because it exists often overrides the need to ask questions about the benefits to be derived from it.

THE RESOLUTION OF CONFLICTS

The conflict between women, faced with such attitudes, and those caring for their health cannot be resolved unless doctors are willing to accept change without feeling threatened; to value time given for discussion without watching the clock; to listen without feeling the need to talk and advise; to continue questioning medical attitudes and actions; to share the choices and decisions with those whose bodies are concerned; and to give back responsibility for health to individuals. None of these changes in attitude can be realized unless doctors are willing to discuss the issues in public and particularly with consumers. It is also vital that consumers should actively determine needs and how to share problems and cooperate in measuring the acceptability and effectiveness of the chosen methods.

Community health councils provide an obvious and welcome channel of communication between the medical profession and the consumers. It is to be hoped that, in time, the effectiveness and influence of these councils will increase. Sample survey techniques as used in market research, commerce and politics could be adapted to provide information rapidly about health needs, the methods used, and their success. Such surveys should be designed by the appropriate non-medical experts for specific, well-defined narrow objectives, and so designed that they could be repeated at intervals to follow the change, to assess the need for further change and to determine the acceptability of the change to the consumer. Doctors should not be the only people to interpret the results of such surveys.

Finally, the emergence of women's self-help groups is another expression of present conflicts in the provision of health services. But these self-help groups also give us hope that we may find new models of health care. As a doctor I find that the needs expressed by women in self-help groups and the methods that they are using in caring for each other provide me with a great deal of knowledge and insight. In no way do I wish to modify their activities, since this would in my opinion hinder the development by women themselves of new ways to meet their health needs and to resolve the conflicts arising from clashes with the paternalistic attitudes of the medical profession.

Discussion

Bridger: The term which many of us would give to the relationship of the doctor with the self-help groups is counselling.

Abercrombie: But Dr Huntingford said that he has no role.

Bridger: But then he defined it: Dr Huntingford, even if you had no role, you had a function.

Huntingford: No, at the moment I have not been given a role—my role is to listen. I am being used, for instance, as a shopkeeper, partly because I can obtain things which women want but cannot get. I then provide it and say that I would be interested to hear what happens.

Guz: What are the implications of rejecting the role of the doctor as the leader of the team?

Huntingford: I am unable to answer questions such as, what do you like done in this situation? It leads to tensions and anxieties amongst my junior staff. I regret that for their sakes, but I am not going to stop rejecting the role of doctor; my junior colleagues must come to terms with their own anxieties.

Guz: I don't understand why you have taken up this position. I accept it as a point of view, with which I don't have much empathy.

Huntingford: Most of my actions are empirical. Most of what one does in obstetrics and gynaecology is not based on irrefutable evidence. Because the woman has been left out of the decision, I want to hand the decision-making process back to her, and therefore I feel that I cannot lead the team as I have nothing to say to them.

Tait: I think you underestimate the extent to which most of us and most patients need boundaries and I suspect that you need them more than you imagine. It is not fair to remove accepted boundaries unless you are prepared to educate people to work in new frameworks and for a long time many patients will need frameworks. We shall never be able to make this an over-the-board decision. The clinician must decide how much responsibility his patient can have.

Huntingford: I disagree; this is the hardest criticism which I have to receive, but I don't accept it because, without starting to do what I do, one cannot continue the process of informing and giving back responsibility. The whole process informs and teaches people. We are being as judgemental in saying that people want boundaries as we were in refraining from telling a patient that he has cancer. It is only an extension of our previous attitude. Giving away responsibility is an extremely time-consuming process.

Weir: In giving away responsibility, you provide patients with information. Is the information often the admission of your empiricism and inability to give advice and information? Do you do this generally?

Huntingford: Yes.

Weir: This must cause a great deal of distress.

Huntingford: I hope it doesn't. Possibly it does, but I cannot judge; others must do so. Obviously, I do not enjoy other people's distress (although I personally enjoy being unhappy, as I have mentioned). I would not continue the experiment (which I don't regard as an experiment) if I felt that I was not justified. I find myself equally at home with my present attitude as when I was following what my teachers had taught me to do.

Bickerton: Where do midwives fit into your scheme?

Huntingford: I try to impart the same attitudes to them. It creates problems.

Paine: First, I must applaud Dr Huntingford; his is a most refreshing view of the doctor–patient relationship. In connection with 'patient-centred' health care teams, it is perhaps relevant that the managers in the reorganized health service seem to be saying that, in the consensus management teams, we can have certain decision-making bodies which have no leader.

Is not the cycle of deprivation in which those who most need the care get least more tied up with education and the ability that people acquire of how to manipulate the system rather than with private practice? The reason that the National Health Service does not have the same standards as private practice is merely a matter of time. In the UK, the health of the population of over 50 million is looked after by the one million who work in the National Health Service. What limits the service they can give is the time at their disposal. If every patient is to take up more of his doctor's time we shall need many more doctors and supporting staff. How many more can we afford in order to obtain what we, as patients, may want?

Huntingford: We don't need more health professionals. I have learnt much from my experience in Asia. In Indonesia there is one nurse for about 40 000 people. The Ministry of Health then decided that one nurse should look after 2000 people. Obviously, there were not enough nurses available but we found that a nurse working within a community was rapidly able to mobilize the neighbouring villages so that in practice she was dealing with about 10 000 people. If she did not deprive those people of their traditional medicine and if she mobilized the villagers to go out and find the expertise they needed (e.g. to produce a water supply, latrines, and to get rid of their rubbish), she was spared these tasks and was then able to hold a surgery in the village square. It is not the number of skilled professionals that is important but the way in which the people around are mobilized. For this reason, self-help groups can be so important; there are many tasks that they want to take on and can do extremely well, for instance, abortion.

Roy: This is similar to my perturbation, possibly as a consequence of service overseas, about where our traditional training has led us and doubts about whether doctors are doing any good for patients. I expect, however, that we shall go through a period of self-doubt to a new confidence, which will then support and refresh us until we reach a further episode of self-doubt. In regard to the training of the younger doctors, I agree with you; specialist training could easily be reduced to four or five years, with more appropriate certification as in North America, Europe, South Africa and Australia. But, as a member of an Examination Committee of a Royal College I know that such a suggestion would meet great opposition, some of this opposition being derived from concern about College income which is so closely related to the present system of training and examination.

Huntingford: That's what I am attacking.

Roy: What is your solution—a shortened training period? Will our successors be able to evolve their philosophy as they go along rather than having to face periods of self-doubt at spaced intervals?

Bridger: Your comment about the opposition in a Royal College is exactly the claim that Dr Huntingford made for the other kinds of health forms in the village complexes in Indonesia: let them keep what they have at the moment and then later move through to something else. This means allowing boundaries to remain for a time.

Lucas: To clarify the concept of total consumer control, let us suppose that, for example, a healthy woman asks you, for private reasons that she does not want to discuss, to remove her uterus and amputate her breasts. What would your response be?

Huntingford: I would say, no; because I am not willing to mutilate somebody and subject her to a risk (inherent in both operations) unless she has fully weighed the risks and the reasons (which she may have done, but will not allow me to know). Your example is too extreme for me to be able to face; however, I have faced a similar request for sterilization and accepted it. The difference between the two requests is that I can understand the reason for sterilization. I have also removed a uterus on request, because I recognized an unexpressed problem of homosexuality. Such situations arise relatively infrequently: I have never been faced with a demand to do something without any sort of explanation. Women will share their reasons for wanting an operation when they meet a receptive attitude. For instance, I have never yet heard a request for abortion that was to me unreasonable.

Lucas: So there is a boundary to your concept of consumer control?

Huntingford: Yes; it is, how far can I go?

Arie: I can only go along with your view part of the way, because our duty to do the best for people who come to us for help seems to preclude such a categorical stand. Abortion is a relatively simple issue. But how does one deal with a patient whose judgement is impaired? An extreme instance, which is common in my work, is the demented and psychotically depressed patient. The easy way out is to say that nobody should be treated against their will;

the world would be very different if things were as simple as that! Sometimes the doctor has to follow the difficult way and do what he believes the patient would want if his judgement were not impaired—to act for the patient. Somewhere in the system there must be provision for treating people against their will or for refusing to do what patients ask of one. Dr Lucas' example might be extreme, but that kind of request in plastic surgery is commonplace—people ask for their noses to be changed, for instance. Just as we ask scientists to be socially responsible, so surely doctors have similar obligations with their skills; they cannot make them available unthinkingly, on demand. The doctor cannot abdicate his responsibility in these things (even if he goes, as I do, a great part of the way with you).

Levitt: Community health councils have recently been asked to comment on policy about sterilization of children under 16. That is an extremely difficult issue to learn about and, although one may have an opinion about it, not much information is available for the consumers. It is important that consumers know how to get information on a great range of issues so that they can be good consumers (good for themselves). If the professionals know where the sources of information are, they should share their knowledge.

Huntingford: Information should be made readily available in an assimilable form but often it cannot be. That does not negate the validity of the consumer's opinion. Gut reactions are very important; we are not rational people, we make emotional and irrational decisions and statements. So opinions are important when they are added together to give 'rounded' opinion. One has then to balance what the whole spectrum of opinion means for individuals. It brings me back to what Dr Arie was saying; obviously, I am polarizing the situation in order to try to understand what I am saying and to try to put over a point. If I am compromised in some of my statements, you would not be able to help me know where I still have conflicts. You have pointed to them and I need to be faced with them. Whether I will ever get beyond those boundaries, I am not sure, but I want to. I accept other people's need for boundaries, but the boundaries can be farther away from ourselves than many of us will allow.

Bridger: As Robert Frost wrote in his poem *Mending Wall* (which I recommend): 'good fences make good neighbours'.

Reference

[1] ABERCROMBIE, M. L. J. (1976) The difficulties of changing, in *This volume*, pp. 3–11

General discussion II

Themes for exploration emerging from papers and discussions

These themes were collected by the group and are a synopsis of the major topics of discussion. Apart from some regrouping they are recorded here without alteration.

SUBJECTS NEEDING REDEFINITION

UK health needs

Relationships of 'committees' in the National Health Service (Department of Health and Social Security and other tiers)

Relationships of personnel in the National Health Service (professional, management, patient) (see ref. 1)

Boundaries between 'committees', implications for taking decisions and policy making

PROBLEMS ASSOCIATED WITH CHANGE

Conflict, stress and anxiety

Transitions and their management (for example, participation means: new responsibilities and changing roles; ways of working out not only how to give away responsibility but also how responsibility can be accepted)

Society (changing values affecting changes in health needs and services)

EXAMPLES OF CONFLICTS AND STRESSES

Task—role

Flexibility—rigidity (of role, e.g. professional attitudes)

Community—hospital

Long-term—short-term

Prevention—cure

Open society—closed system

Benefit—cost

Needs (perceived)—resources (available)

EDUCATION

Professional retraining (learning, unlearning, relearning)
Undergraduate training, selection
Recruitment of staff

CONSUMER

Patient as person (respect for individual, sacrosanctity of doctor/patient rela-
    tionship)
Patient as partner/expert
Use of community health councils as partners/experts
Women and their health

TEAMWORK

Interdependent needs
Community health councils
Commitment (participation involves responsibility)

GOALS

Commitment
Integration of different parts of the National Health Service (community
    hospitals, regional hospitals, academic departments, university hospitals)
Operational research (scientific approach to problems)
Community, administrative and professional development
Extension of hospital into community

Roy: Mr Bridger, are you in favour of leadership?

Bridger: Functional leadership, yes; that is to say, leadership that arises
from within or that is assigned according to the character of the task and the
resources in the group.

Roy: So, all groups must have or will produce a leader?

Bridger: We must distinguish between leadership and a leader. The latter
suggests that the group is assigned or elects (say) someone to have the role at
all times—whatever the situation in the group. Leadership is a function which
might be exercised by different members of the group at different times depending on the situation and the task at a given time. It allows an individual to give

the relevant lead. It raises the question, for example, of whether the doctor should be the leader of the team all the time as distinct from being so when appropriate to a particular task. There may well be a case for someone to exercise the role of chairman (as in this symposium) or manager—but his *leadership function* should only come into play when it is thought relevant. All too often it may be practised inappropriately and cause those concerned to feel that they are being bull-dozed or directed to suit the person in the *leader role,* who in their eyes is exercising his *function of leadership* wrongly.[2] In a further example which applies here too, the chairman or manager may have the role and be concerned with keeping an eye on the various objectives, while enabling others to express their leadership either through the content of the tasks ahead or through changing the way the group is operating internally.

For instance, consider our list of themes; several overlap. These are themes which have been extracted from what we are actually doing. If we were going to tackle any of these themes and make some concrete suggestions for another meeting, what kind of tasks would we want to formulate? We have been exploring some of the developments, issues, forces, factors and problems that are encouraging and bothering us. Now we move to the point where we can select some options and make some choices about where to explore at greater depth, and find out who then would want, and be appropriate, to take part in such a follow-up experience.

Roy: We are talking about two aspects of change: what we think might happen through change and what we would like to see happen through change. The changes that we are considering are changes in attitudes, and reallocation and rethinking of the tasks we do.

Bridger: Some of these could apply to ourselves.

Roy: Therefore, we are considering how change can be brought about and how, away from this symposium, we can be brought into a relationship with the people who like us want to change attitudes and tasks. One solution will be medical advisory committees and the like, which we rather despise and about which we are disturbed. We come back to the framework, both formal and informal; we have not talked about informal contacts to any extent but if we talk too much about them they might become formal.

Paine: Those sorts of feelings lie behind the heading about redefinition of UK health needs.

If we are to have any hope of coming to practicalities in the new, now formalized, structure of the health service, this will be done by bodies that have been mentioned by Dr Russell (p. 28) and Miss Levitt (p. 55), namely the health care planning teams. These are supposed to define the needs of their districts and areas. They are interprofessional but do not contain (anyway as yet) patients or consumer representatives—hence the sub-heading about the role of consumer as expert. Nevertheless, we pin our faith on these planning teams in the formal structure so that we can balance needs and resources more effectively.

Roy: Again I ask, if a tier in the reorganized health service must disappear, what are we going to do about it? If it is so important, can we afford to wait? How can we get rid of it with as little trauma as possible?

Bridger: Speaking now personally and not as chairman, why not change the relationship between the Department of Health and Social Security and the rest of the National Health Service so that what is now the Region becomes a functional advisory agency covering the boundary between the Department and the rest? Extension of the Department into the health service itself was avoided in the reorganization despite the verbal theoretical promise about devolution and delegation of authority.

Weir: I don't mean to be unduly cynical but the only tier we can do away with is the Department of Health and Social Security or, in Scotland, the Scottish Home and Health Department (there is a difference between the administration in Scotland and in England and Wales). Doing away with the intermediate tier leads to more central control, not less. We need scope to make the services that we are providing relevant to the community.

Bridger: But you are making the assumption that the Department cannot be altered. You may be right!

Hockey: Many of the crucial issues are not directly related to reorganization in the health service. Even though we have problems with bureaucracy, we ought to identify more clearly how we could meet our patients' needs better if the service were reorganized differently or had not been reorganized in the way it has. Most of the papers we have heard have been unrelated to the structure of the health service.

Tait: The last few discussions have been tense and emotionally charged. We talked and thought a lot about dying, how to cope with dying, and it seemed in a way that we were talking about the dying of something as well as of patients: the dying of the health service perhaps, or the dying of the authoritarian doctor, the 'magician' doctor, as the central force in the health service, which he can no longer be. And then we began to think of a rebirth through a partnership with the community. Dr Huntingford pushed this as far as he could to challenge us. The hope for the future coming out of this struggling session seems to be that, if we can learn how to build this partnership and make the community grow to the stature of its tasks, then we may create a new kind of medical care system.

Russell: The power base is changing, and we must know how far the public can tolerate the changes we are discussing before we can advance with the other shifts in power base: from hospital to community (in terms of services), from doctors to other professions, etc.

Abercrombie: This is a shifting area. There are different thresholds which at different times are mobile. In our work with students in groups, with the aim of helping them to become autonomous (i.e. the equivalent of the community taking over), we have noticed that after a few intensive discussions on videotapes of their classes they begin to realize that they could run the group themselves. If the change is not too great, the movement will be in the right direction and will gain strength. One cannot define the impact of change in a static way; the degree of change we can tolerate now differs from the amount we could learn to tolerate in the future.

Levitt: Although that sounds right, how does one make that particular? In general, the community will discover its strength by dealing with particular issues. It is not clear from what you say how they can respond.

Bridger: Aren't we trying here now? I have not adopted the traditional role of chairman in relation to this group and its tasks. This group also has innovated and experimented with different approaches in discussion. Everyone has been taking part.

Knox: We tend to make a distinction between 'us' in the National Health Service and 'them' in the community but we should be saying that there is an organization called the health service which is an institution of the community. We should not so much be advocating community participation as accepting the idea of community *control*—but so many of our definitions and practices of participation exclude such a possibility. Elsewhere[3] I have described how organizations with traditional hierarchical structures can adapt themselves to 'accept' some democratic or participatory function, and that the analogy of an 'Indian Reservation' for tamed militants may be nearer the truth than many of us would care to admit. Bailey[4] has suggested that the intellectual interests defended are those which are rooted in a pluralist view of democracy, and that the views of bureaucracy and decision-making are 'essentially subsidiary to the theory that "fair" representation leads to decisions which can be accommodated by a homogenous and consensual society'. Opportunities and mechanisms of participation may unfortunately supply props to such a value system by presenting the system as not only being flexible and democratic but also conveying the sense that it has a social commitment and idealism coupled with a close identification with the community and its needs. Without control, the community may only get at most education and at least a pretence at consultation.

Huntingford: These abstract discussions have been necessary but now we need to be practical. The suggested headings for further discussion fall into two groups; both provide a starting point for discussion. I would certainly want to start without any assumptions and ask how we define health needs.

Elliott: Another issue is *needs* contrasted with *wants*; wants are sometimes assumed to be needs. There are sometimes demands on a health service which are wants and which might not be recognized by the bureaucracy as needs.

Huntingford: This would come clear from detailed consideration. Can any of the other headings be amalgamated to produce a more manageable list?

Arie: Many are concerned with conflict and polarization: such as the conflict between perceived need, and what is available; and false polarities, such as 'the hospital' and 'the community'. Above all, these days, we find that having defined needs we lack the resources for meeting them. How do we cope with that and tolerate it and make it most just?

Roy: Needs, wants and tasks change from year to year. How can we have a system that automatically resolves the conflicts which arise from the polarities that exist at present and will subsequently be formed?

Arie: Some by their nature seem to be unresolvable. How do we live with unresolved conflicts?

Roy: Can we resolve them or accommodate them?

Tait: The structure poses a problem; unless we liberate the constraints (guidelines) at some level we cannot rediscover ways ahead; we cannot begin the new partnership with the client. At the moment the discussion is stiff because while there is a need to try new things we cannot in practice do anything, or so it seems.

Bridger: When speaking of conflict and polarization we need to distinguish these more extreme positions from that in which we often find ourselves when we try to reconcile, or balance and optimize, certain aims, outlooks or values.

Dr Huntingford (pp. 157–161) mentioned the difficulties associated with the conflicts facing women at present when they have so many forces and factors to reconcile in deciding, for example, whether to have a hysterectomy. Is this not an instance of the price a person pays for the freedom gained in coming out of a past role? If one assumes an environment in which certain values exist from which there is no escape (the attitude of the church, of the government, of society to the role of women in the home etc.) then the step to be taken or even the questioning of whether something happens tends not to get explored. In such a case, the social norm of authority, in the shape of the doctor, decides. The individual may, depending on many circumstances, suffer intrapersonal stress or be glad to have someone else decide. The values, norms, culture, conventions all play their part to varying degrees in any society. But the moment the climate encourages or allows these values to begin changing or the institutions embodying the establishment are themselves affected by the changes, boundaries are lowered—other opportunities, potential freedoms and possibilities arise. But with the freedoms, the responsibilities and decisions deriving from them move from society, its established institutions and recognized 'authorities' to the individuals, groups and professions concerned. By the same token, the doctor, the nurse and so on find personal and role boundaries extended. As a result they become involved in dealing with most (if not all) of the themes on our list. Then, perhaps, the freedoms and powers have that double-edged effect. The scope is fine so long as it does not entail continually making decisions. We find increasingly that people want to participate; the problem of shared responsibility that goes with participation has, however, not been bargained for. This issue of greater sharing of responsibilities with increased participation implies a more interdependent set of relationships with professional and other colleagues, at various levels. Much more of our work also demands greater multidisciplinary capability, and this intensifies our need for competence in coping with increased interdependence.

To return to my original comment on the distinction and effects of a relatively stable environment with its corresponding norms and values compared with that of a relatively unstable, uncertain and complex one, we may be required to work, in this latter situation, in a way approaching what Dr Huntingford described as having 'no boundaries'. But as there are always limits to communication, freedoms and scope, we need to learn where the boundaries of our more 'open system' are. With the disadvantages and constraints of the past we had a clearer picture of 'our place' in the order of things; today we have, among other problems, that of identity ('boundary'). This is as true for doctor, nurse and so on as it is for other roles and professions in society. In addition to the importance of improving our competence in interdependent working we also need to learn how to review our freedoms and constraints with others, and measure them against our own and others' expectations. Many features that we are discussing are those which derive from making sense and endeavouring to regulate (control) our own activities and objectives in a total setting of change. The change that has been underestimated is the way in which any part of a system interacts, affects and is affected by other parts, including an increasing lack of predictability in our various environments. This, to me, is what Escher's work is about; one of his most striking pictures is 'Metamorphosis'. Like Dr Abercrombie, I find his work most impressive and interpretative—an artistic combination of thought and cross-cultural change. It seemed that Escher was putting on canvas what I have tried to do at the Tavistock Institute.

Huntingford: Are you suggesting that it would be more appropriate to try to define what sort of transition we are passing through rather than to define needs at the moment, because that is impossible?

Bridger: Dr Beckhard referred to certain agencies that were being developed to facilitate relationships between diverse bodies and functions. Can some of the issues which we have discussed help us to understand and change the past without, at the same time, letting us assume that we have arrived in the future too fast? What kind of agencies do we need to deal with the diverse problems and certain polarities each of us has in his or her field?

The capacity to tolerate uncertainty around us and to handle many frames of reference in our thinking is rare; yet, increasingly, these attributes are required in developing our interdependence for effective outcomes.

Hockey: Interdependence creates a live organism with potential for growth and development. The phrase 'tolerating change' has connotations of having to cope with things, and I want to feel that we can use or direct change, or see the potential of change for better patient care.

Tait: Is there a special difficulty for us? We think as doctors and we are now talking about problems; we transfer the problems into pathology and we then feel especially responsible for solving them medically. I feel that I am supposed to go out with a 'problem-solving' penicillin and cure everything. Perhaps we have to learn to accept terminal illnesses about which we can do nothing— terminal illnesses of some kinds of medicine as well as of patients.

Bridger: The penicillin has not taken over your previous relationship with the patient; you are still in contact with the patient. How do you manage the three elements—you, the patient and the penicillin—as distinct from what you did in the past? In some other cases, however, the penicillin may have taken over: where doling out penicillin is felt to be all that is necessary and the patient, as a person, is left out. In contrast to what we are saying about the patient as a person, many general practitioners complain that all many people want is the prescription.

Roy: It is extremely unlikely that we shall move from instability to stability in isolation from what is happening elsewhere in society. How important is it that we should understand the general picture of society before we can hope to meet the problems of the present phase of instability?

Bridger: We have now met as discussants and contributors. In so doing we found a *raison d'être* related to our list of themes and our thoughts on them. If now, at the end of the symposium, we were to approach the organizers at the Ciba Foundation and say that we had something to offer, what would it be and how would we do it? We could leave here feeling that we have a mass of good material, that we have teased certain problems out, raised issues, many of which are covered by the headings we assembled.

Roy: It worries me that we still consider the community as only the people who come to us as patients. The instability that we feel may also be the instability that makes people become terrorists and the instability that is diffused throughout our society. I cannot see the health service suddenly becoming tranquil and organized and evolving gently and peacefully unless all the other components of society change at the same time.

Russell: Presumably there must be many others who are aware of these problems and who are also making small steps to cross the barriers we have mentioned.

At a smaller and more personal level than the structure of health services, we may be able to test the general hypothesis that we have put forward. A smaller scale makes it more comprehensible to most of us and we can see the kinds of changes that we are testing more easily than if we were to take on a big issue in one step.

McClymont: I agree. These discussions seem to have generated a sense of powerlessness to change the total structure. If we hypothesize all night about transforming the administrative structure of the health service, we won't get anywhere! We must develop some of the ideas on consumer participation and interprofessional cooperation in our own spheres of activity.

Birley: Can we put our discussion in the context of Popper's *Open Society*,[5] and his plea for piecemeal solutions rather than total ones? It is a humbler approach. Illich's *Medical Nemesis*[6] (with which I disagree profoundly) has the value of pointing out the fate of the proud. In talking about solutions, we are inclined to be rather puffed up. It is helpful to assume that most of us working in the health service are rather stupid and so are our patients and 'the community'. If we manage to make a third-rate system work, we shall be doing well. And, like a third-division football club, we might gain promotion. As in football, the club needs continuous management to keep up. There are no 'solutions' that work over any length of time. If we create a total system, then we also create terrorists, because only terrorism can destroy a total system. Only one remark here got me reaching for my gun, and that was when Dr Weir said that, unless we are *completely clear* about our roles, we will never make progress. That is a 'totalitarian' statement—what Popper might call a Platonic one—and, of course, all Scotsmen are Platonists! We have been enjoying the privilege of rather grandiose discussions in a beautiful classical building, but we can't be Humphrey Reptons or Capability Browns. We have got to get back to our allotments and try to alter our little patches where necessary, encourage the promising lines, and try out new ones if we can.

Roy: The instability has set in imperceptibly. We are now seeking ways in which we could imperceptibly begin to push the tide back again.

Tait: A sort of intermediate technology of change.

Birley: Meanwhile we are in danger of having a total system imposed on us.

Bridger: With your 'allotments' I want to couple Miss Hockey's observation (p. 63) that 'problems should be seen as seed beds for progress rather than frustration' and that they should be used in that way to stimulate change. Furthermore, Dr Russell was right to add that progress will only be little by little. We must now, in view of what we have discussed, reappraise our own allotments and then, in the future, compare our experiences, supplementing what we have shared in this symposium by exploring issues we have faced up to now.

Weir: But this will not resolve the problems that most people face in the health service because, as you pointed out, there are so few people who can tolerate conflict and change in the way that has been described. That is why I stress that unless people define their roles—what they see as their functions— we cannot move to this situation, because people can only realize the needs of others in relation to their own expectations.

Birley: With respect to the conflict between task and role, a task is easier to define, but it may turn out that the task can be done with fewer people. That is threatening, and it is what may be happening in various sections of the health service.

Bridger: The closer we get to a particular task, on our own allotments, the less easy it will be to share with everybody else later. We will also need, therefore, to think of ways in which we can enable others to understand and grow the 'seeds' or 'cuttings' we offer from our 'allotments'. In this respect our efforts, successful or unsuccessful, will all be valuable as contributions.

Arie: Dr Birley's comments attract me, coming as I do from an impoverished sector of the health service and a large poor mental hospital—poor in fabric and in resources. In the pleasant hospitality of the Ciba Foundation, we talk objectively about the hideously tatty, irrational and unintelligent situations in which we work. But even to be able to work at all is a privilege at a time when 1 250 000 (and more) people are unemployed and none of us can be sure that we shall be drawing our salaries in six months' time. At the same time medical colleagues have lately been turning away patients, and threatening the moral base of our profession. Meanwhile, we have to operate a day-to-day 'rationing' of our service at the interface with the public, but with no publicly declared criteria for the rationing. This may make unreal such questions as we have been debating—'Will I perform the abortion simply because the woman wants it?' The issue that is likely to be forced on us is 'How can I do the operation when I have too few beds, too few staff, no safe operating theatres?' I am constantly confronted by obviously needy situations which I cannot meet. These are my everyday working realities to which I shall return.

McClymont: But that is the same dilemma that everybody else has been raising.

Huntingford: We return to the allotment proposition—a consideration of what is practical and tangible comes next. My attitudes did not change rationally, but I now accept the changes and attempt to use them to solve a problem.

Bridger: Instead of communicating and arguing intellectually about a problem we want others to join us in looking at it, how we considered it, the decisions and actions we took and, then, to help us explore it a bit more. Each of us is also a consumer.

Roberts: I like the allotment idea. Two 'seeds' have particularly interested me. First, the notion that we could study, objectively, ways in which the consumer can be involved in decisions about the provision of health care. Screening may be a suitable area to examine; a sample of consumers could be given information about the benefits and costs of screening for (say) neural tube defects, or hypertension, and their views on the need for either of these services analysed. The second seed that may be worth cultivating is the effect of voluntary, community-based, self-help groups on the quality of life of the disadvantaged, such as those suffering from a stroke who were receiving traditional care. The support of self-help groups could be compared with those who had access only to traditional care.

Huntingford: Are we not creating another job for ourselves at the moment?

Russell: We are not creating more work but are analysing more clearly from a common base what we are trying to solve. Our targets and methods may differ but the principles of analysis are the same.

Bridger: A most important point; we have been searching around in this last discussion, sometimes moving into difficult areas. Dr Birley has helped us by bringing in not just a metaphor but the idea of the allotment which has been expanded and adopted in various ways.

Arie: Would it focus our sights if we thought of any next phase with the idea of this group giving evidence to the Royal Commission, using the evidence from our own work? That might act as a discipline but, on the other hand, we might be able to do something more useful.

Bridger: First the allotment, then the implications for the Royal Commission.

We have shared much. Any other group would have to start all over again and work through to this stage. We have coped with our established tolerances and differences and can now build on a set of working relationships. In agreeing to a follow-up we are testing our commitment. I wish everyone well on their allotments and look forward to meeting you all on 'Harvest Day'.

References

[1] MANNING, C. (1974) *The Reorganised National Health Service*, Health and Social Service Journal, London
[2] SELZNIK, P. (1957) *Leadership in Administration*, Harper & Row, London
[3] KNOX, J.J. (1974) *Citizen Participation in Health Care—some comparisons in two cultures.* Presentation to the Smithsonian Institution and Fellows of the Woodrow Wilson International Center for Scholars (Series on Voluntarism), Washington D.C.
[4] BAILEY, J. (1957) *Social Theory for Planning*, Routledge and Kegan Paul, London
[5] POPPER, K.R. (1962) *Open Society and its Enemies*, Routledge and Kegan Paul, London
[6] ILLICH, I. (1975) *Medical Nemesis, The Expropriation of Health*, Calder & Boyars, London

Biographies of the participants

M. L. J. ABERCROMBIE, a biologist, has worked mostly at University College London on selection and education of medical and architectural students and is especially interested in perception, reasoning, communication and small group work. Her publications include *The Anatomy of Judgment* (1960); *Perceptual and Visuomotor Disorders in Cerebral Palsy* (1964); *Aims and Techniques of Group Teaching* (1970).

TOM ARIE is chiefly interested in the organization and functions of health and social services, and in the education and job-satisfaction of staff. Lately he has been a member of government working parties on social services policy and of the Central Council for Education and Training in Social Work. His main work is in his psychiatric unit for old people in East London, where he is Consultant Psychiatrist at Goodmayes Hospital, and he is also Honorary Senior Lecturer in Psychiatry at University College Hospital Medical School.

HOWARD BADERMAN, born in 1934, is Consultant Physician in Charge of Accident and Emergency Services at University College Hospital, London. He was Senior Registrar in medical administration at University College Hospital between 1968 and 1970 with full-time attachment to one of the then London Metropolitan Regional Hospital Boards and has worked on various committees at the Department of Health in London. He has made special study of admission procedures, waiting list control and bed state management in hospitals on behalf of the King Edward's Hospital Fund for London. He is now Secretary to the Specialist Advisory Committee on Accident and Emergency Medicine to the Joint Committee on Higher Medical and Surgical Training of the Royal Colleges of Physicians and Surgeons in London.

RICHARD BECKHARD is adjunct professor of management at the Sloan School of Management at Massachusetts Institute of Technology, Director of Richard Beckhard Associates in New York, and consultant to the Association of American Medical Colleges on their management advancement program. He is doing research on applications of management to education of health workers and organization of health delivery systems. His publications include, *Organization Development: Strategies & Models*, *Strategies For Large System Change*, *Making Health Teams Work*,

179

Organizational Issues in the Team Delivery of Comprehensive Health Care, The Education of the Health Care Team—What's It All About.

MAVIS BICKERTON is Senior Nursing Officer (Community), Hertfordshire Area Health Authority. She was formerly a Nursing Officer (Health Visiting) for the Bedfordshire Area Health Authority. She gained her health visiting experience in group attachment with Berkshire County Council, Cheshire County Council and Stockport Area Health Authority. She has other nursing experience in Family Planning and in a Government Rehabilitation Medical Unit. She is currently Health Visitor representative on the Court Committee of the Department of Health and Social Security.

J.L.T. BIRLEY, born in 1928, is Dean of the Institute of Psychiatry and Consultant to Bethlem Royal and Maudsley Hospital. He has done research in social psychiatry, and is particularly interested in the development of local psychiatric services.

HAROLD BRIDGER is a founder member of the Tavistock Institute of Human Relations where he is currently concerned with action-research and training in the field of organizational change and career development. A significant part of his work is international and he is a founder member and Secretary General of the European Institute for Transnational Studies in Group and Organizational Development. He is particularly interested in the patterns of change in professions and is a member of a London Area Health Authority.

RICHARD CARTER was trained as a chemist and did research in organic chemistry at the University of Bristol. He took up operational research in 1966 and has worked for several bodies in the public sector. Since 1971 he has been a principal scientific officer in the Operational Research Service of the Department of Health and Social Security, with particular interest in the applications of operational research in primary health care.

KATHERINE ELLIOTT is Assistant Director of the Ciba Foundation. She has worked in paediatrics and obstetrics in England and India. She has organized several Ciba Ciba Foundation symposia, including *The Family and its Future, Teamwork for World Health, Human Rights in Health, Size at Birth* and *Health and Industrial Growth* and is Chairman of the Intermediate Technology Group's rural health panel. She is the author of two annotated bibliographies and several articles on the role of auxiliaries in health care.

ELSIE GOLLAN, born in 1914, is Administrative Secretary, Caversham Group Practice, Kentish Town Health Centre.

ROY GOULSTON has for some years been a general practitioner in a London group practice but originally comes from Sydney, Australia. As Course Organizer for general practitioner teachers he is closely involved with postgraduate training.

ABRAHAM GUZ, born in 1929, has a personal Chair in Medicine at Charing Cross Hospital Medical School, University of London. He has worked mainly in the area of the neurophysiology of lung reflexes, the analysis of mechanisms of dyspnoea, and the assessment of cardiac performance. He was Secretary of the Medical Research Society 1968–1973.

LISBETH HOCKEY is a qualified nurse, midwife, district nurse and health visitor with a B.Sc. in Economics. After wide practical, administrative and teaching experience in various fields of nursing she became involved in nursing research and published a series of research reports on nursing issues. She has been Director of the Nursing Research Unit in the University of Edinburgh since 1971.

PETER J. HUNTINGFORD, born in 1929, is Professor of Clinical Obstetrics and Gynaecoogy in the Joint Academic Unit of Obstetrics, Gynaecology and Reproductive Physiology of the University of London at St. Bartholomew's Hospital and the London Hospital Medical Colleges. He was previously Professor of Obstetrics and Gynaecology at St. Mary's Hospital Medical School, Paddington. Between these two appointments he served with the World Health Organization as Regional Adviser in Maternal and Child Health to the South-East Asia Regional Office, New Delhi, and later in field projects in Thailand and Indonesia.

GRAHAM JOYSON, born and educated in Lancashire, is at present the Superintendent of Nursing of the Royal Marsden Hospital, London and Sutton, a member of the Education Panel of the South West Thames Regional Cancer Council and a member of The Joint Board of Clinical Nursing Studies. He is Director of Nursing designate at the Royal Melbourne Hospital, Victoria, Australia.

JULIAN J. KNOX is Secretary of Islington Community Health Council. He has been Director of the Institute for Social Research, London, and held posts at the Sorbonne, Paris, on the International Social Science Council of UNESCO; in the Tavistock Institute for Human Relations, at Yale University School of Medicine, and Georgetown University. He was a program consultant to the US Department of Health Education & Welfare, Health Services Administration. He is a founding member of INTERPLAN, Paris. His principal interest is the development of methodologies for community participation in planning and decision-making with special reference to contributions from the social and behavioural sciences.

RUTH LEVITT, born in 1950, is editor of *CHC NEWS*—an information bulletin/newsletter for community health councils and was Project Consultant, Charing Cross Hospital, before that. She is the author of *The Reorganized National Health Service* and is a CHC member.

C.J. LUCAS is Director and Psychiatric Adviser of the Health Centre, University College London. After training in general medicine, psychiatry and psychiatric research, he took up his present post in 1959. His main interests are psychotherapy in a university context and problems of work difficulty on which he has published several papers.

MARY E. MCCLYMONT is Principal Lecturer in Health Studies at Stevenage College, Hertfordshire. She has worked mainly in community health nursing and nursing education but was Nurse Tutor at University College Hospital, Ibadan, Nigeria, and Education Officer at Queen's Institute of District Nursing, London.

LESLIE H. W. PAINE was awarded a bursary to study hospital administration by the King Edward's Hospital Fund for London in 1950. He was appointed House Governor and Secretary to the Bethlem Royal Hospital and the Maudsley Hospital in 1963, a post he still holds. His publications include *Know Your Hospital*, *What is a Good Hospital*, *N.H.S. and E.E.C.*, *Twenty-Four Talks*, *Coordinating Services for the Mentally Handicapped*. He is also currently Editor of *World Hospitals*, the quarterly journal of the International Hospital Federation.

COLIN ROBERTS, born in 1936 in Birmingham, is Senior Lecturer in Epidemiology, Welsh National School of Medicine, and Consultant Community Physician to the South Glamorgan Area Health Authority (Teaching). His early research was largely concerned with the aetiology of congenital malformations, neuropsychiatric disorders in childhood, and ischaemic heart disease. He is now working mainly on applied research studies in clinical and in community medicine.

DOUGLAS ROY is Professor of Surgery at The Queen's University, Belfast. He held consultant posts in the Western Infirmary, Glasgow, until becoming involved in the establishment of a medical school in Nairobi in 1965. He was appointed Foundation Professor of Surgery in Nairobi in 1968, leaving East Africa in 1972. He became increasingly interested in the relationship of medical schools to the communities they serve and their involvement with the training of all medical workers. He is presently also consultant to the University of Sierra Leone with regard to University involvement in the training of medical auxiliaries.

ELIZABETH M. RUSSELL is Senior Lecturer in Community Medicine, University of Aberdeen. She has worked mainly in general practice and medical administration (Scottish-style). She teaches medical sociology and is concerned with research in rehabilitation and health economics.

I. G. TAIT has been a general practitioner in Suffolk for 16 years. He has taken an active part in the development of programmes of vocational training for general practice in East Anglia and is an Associate Regional Adviser in postgraduate education. During 1971 he was a Nuffield Travelling Fellow and studied the teaching of Behavioural Science in the Medical Schools of North America, and the use of general and family practice for this purpose. He has a particular interest in problem-orientated medical records and in their use in medical education. He has recently been appointed the Jephcott Visiting Professor in general practice to University College Hospital Medical School, an appointment which he will hold during 1976.

ROY D. WEIR is head of the Department of Community Medicine at Aberdeen University and a member of the Grampian Health Board. His interests include epidemiology, computing in medicine, information services, operational research and the organization and evaluation of health care.

Index of contributors

Entries in bold type indicate papers; other entries refer to contributions to discussions

Indexes compiled by William Hill

183

Subject index

185